PRAISE FOR *MUSHROOM ESSENCES*

"Charting new territory and going where no one else has gone before always takes special courage and oversight. Within the realm of vibrational preparations, mushrooms and lichens have hitherto been almost entirely ignored. With his remarkable research, Robert Rogers gifts us with unprecedented insight into a neglected corner of energy medicine. Rogers presents several novel ways of essence preparation, showing his deep and sensitive communion with nature. Detailing the indications and uses of forty-eight new essences backed up with case histories, he poetically weaves together this must-read source of mushroom wisdom."
—**Julia Graves,** author of *The Language of Plants*

"If we are to reach our fullest potential, we must learn about and integrate the shadow. As difficult as this journey can be, we have been provided the means to be supported throughout it: the fungi. Robert Rogers's work with their intelligence in the form of "essences" to augment this challenging journey is a poignant eye-opener—one many of us may not be ready for, but one we dearly need. *Mushroom Essences* provides a valuable toolkit for anyone on the herbal path towards psychospiritual health."
—**James W. Jesso,** author of *True Light Of Darkness*

"Soul connection, transformation, healing the traumatized psyche—these are the purview of mushroom essences. They transmute the dark elements of our injured minds and spirits to experiences and expressions of the authentic, joyous life that is our birthright. They speak healing truths to the body, mind, and spirit without harm or pain. In *Mushroom Essences* Robert Rogers gives us clear knowledge, means, and methods for personal freedom and wholeness."
—**Sandra Dutreau Williams, PhD,** founder and director of Mushrooms for Well Being Foundation

MUSHROOM ESSENCES

Vibrational Healing from the Kingdom Fungi

ROBERT DALE ROGERS, RH (AHG)

Foreword by Willoughby Arevalo

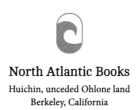

North Atlantic Books
Huichin, unceded Ohlone land
Berkeley, California

Published by
North Atlantic Books
Huichin, unceded Ohlone land
Berkeley, California

Cover photo by Taylor Lockwood
Cover and book design by Howie Severson
Printed in the United States of America

Mushroom Essences: Vibrational Healing from the Kingdom Fungi is sponsored and published by North Atlantic Books, an educational nonprofit based in the unceded Ohlone land Huichin (Berkeley, CA) that collaborates with partners to develop cross-cultural perspectives; nurture holistic views of art, science, the humanities, and healing; and seed personal and global transformation by publishing work on the relationship of body, spirit, and nature.

North Atlantic Books's publications are distributed to the US trade and internationally by Penguin Random House Publishers Services. For further information, visit our website at www.northatlanticbooks.com.

MEDICAL DISCLAIMER: The following information is intended for general information purposes only. Individuals should always see their health care provider before administering any suggestions made in this book. Any application of the material set forth in the following pages is at the reader's discretion and is their sole responsibility.

Library of Congress Cataloging-in-Publication Data
Rogers, Robert Dale, 1950- author.
Mushroom essences : vibrational healing from the kingdom fungi / Robert Dale
  Rogers, RH (AHG) ; foreword by Willoughby Arevalo.
pages cm
Summary: "A guide to the benefits of mushroom essences for mental, emotional, and
  spiritual health"—Provided by publisher.
Includes bibliographical references.
ISBN 978-1-62317-045-5 (print)
1. Essences and essential oils—Therapeutic use. 2. Mushrooms—Therapeutic use.
  3. Medicinal plants. 4. Materia medica, Vegetable. I. Title.
RM666.A68R63 2016
615.9'5296—dc23   2015034902

4 5 6 7 8 9 10 5LP 26 25 24

North Atlantic Books is committed to the protection of our environment. We print on recycled paper whenever possible and partner with printers who strive to use environmentally responsible practices.

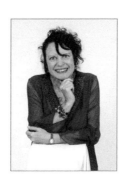

This book is dedicated to my soul mate and love of my life, Laurie Szott-Rogers (pictured). She is the fun gal who makes my life rich and exciting, but also gently nudges against all my shadow sides.

It is a big job.

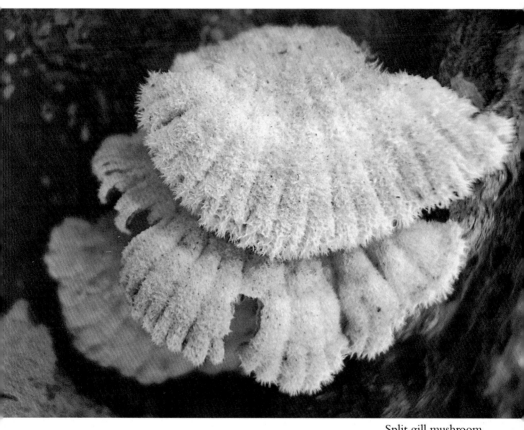

Split gill mushroom

ACKNOWLEDGMENTS

I hardly know where to begin, but I should probably start with thanking a number of remarkable professional and amateur mycologists. If your name is not mentioned here, I apologize in advance. Now, where did I put that bottle of *Hericium* supplements?

From Edmonton, my hometown for the past thirty years, I wish to thank Martin Osis, Bill Richards, Rob Simpson, and other members of the Alberta Mycological Society for their mentorship, friendship, and numerous enjoyable forays.

I wish to thank a number of members of the North American Mycological Society (NAMA), including their support of my few years as chairman of the medicinal mushroom committee.

I owe special thanks to Dr. Solomon Wasser, editor in chief of *The International Journal of Medicinal Mushrooms*. His dedication to research in this area is second to none.

I would also like to thank all the friends and acquaintances I have met at forays over the years, including Paul Stamets, Todd and Doug Elliott, Scott Redhead, Jim Ginns, Paul Kroeger, Larry Evans, Daniel Winkler, Cathy Cripps, John Plischke III, Taylor Lockwood, Tom Volk, and Duane Sept.

Thanks to all the clubs, guilds, and societies that have invited me to speak to their members on the subject of medicinal mushrooms, including the South Vancouver Island Mycological Society (SVIMS), the Georgia Mycological Society, the South Carolina University Mycological Society (SCUMS), the Vancouver Mycological Society, the Mycological Society of San Francisco, SOMA camp, the American Herbalist Guild, and the Horticultural Society of Iceland.

I give special thanks to the Telluride Mushroom Festival, the King Bolete celebration of all things Fungi. Tradd and Olga Cotter, Gary Lincoff, John Holliday, Rebecca Fyfe, Maggie Klinedinst, Art Goodtimes, Daiva Chesonis, Lawrence Millman, Peter McCoy, Enrique Sanchez, and numerous fun gals and fun guys make this an annual highlight of the mushroom season.

I would be remiss if I did not mention my clients and students over the past thirty years who helped me gain insight into a different dimension of mushroom healing.

I offer special thanks to Edward C. Whitmont, Thomas Moore, Sam Keen, Bill Plotkin, José Stevens, Martin Ball, David Richo, and numerous other authors who have offered their insights into the underworld journey toward soul connection.

I am grateful to Doug Reil at North Atlantic Books for his belief and support in the project, and to Erin Wiegand and Nina Pick for painstakingly editing my wandering streams of consciousness. I mean, what else would you expect from an author of mushroom essences?

And many thanks to various photographer friends for sharing pictures for this publication. I enjoy taking my own pictures, but these individuals are in a different league in terms of talent and quality. Thank you.

CONTENTS

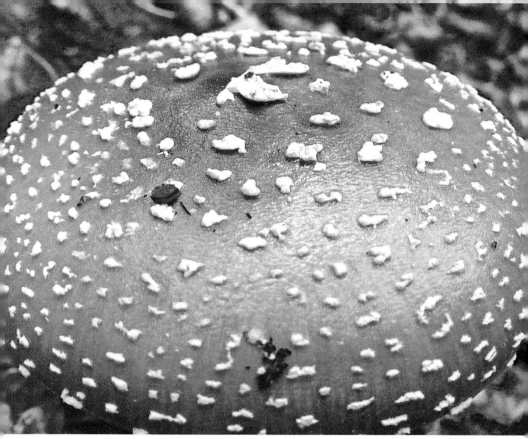

Fly agaric

DISCLAIMER: The following information is intended for general information purposes only. Individuals should always see their health care provider before administering any suggestions made in this book. The suggestions, recipes, and historical information are not meant to replace a medical adviser. The author assumes no liability for unwise or unsafe usage or preparation of mushroom essences by readers of this book. For those interested in using mushroom essences, seek the advice of a professional. Some mushrooms contain deadly poisons. The author and publisher assume no legal responsibility for individuals producing or ingesting essences based on this book.

FOREWORD

Mushrooms have mystified people since ancient times. Their spontaneous appearance has been linked to lightning, deities, supernatural beings, and the excrescences of wild beasts. They seem to embody the magic and mystery of the subterranean world. This magic caught my attention when I was a young child, and mushrooms have been a major passion in my life ever since.

Before I had heard of mushroom essences, I visited an herbalist friend in Arizona who specialized in creating herbal formulas, including flower essences. I asked her about the process of interpreting flower essences. She told me that she listened to the plants through meditation to hear what they had to share with us. I imagined mushrooms could impart their energetics into an essence as well, not knowing that this practice already existed. Having spent much time over the course of my life relating to mushrooms in a mind-frame of study and observation, I was drawn to explore the personalities and vibrational medicines of fungi, but I lacked a mentor to guide me on this journey.

I met Robert Rogers when our paths overlapped on our way to the Telluride Mushroom Festival in 2013. He was invited to present on medicinal mushrooms, and I on fungal sexuality. I felt an immediate connection to him as we spoke about the medicinal, energetic, and sensual properties of mushrooms. I had first encountered his book *The Fungal Pharmacy* a year and a half earlier and had gobbled it up. It presents a holistic perspective on medicinal mushrooms unprecedented in the body of mycological literature, and it remains one of my primary reference materials when researching a mushroom. An aspect of the book that particularly grabbed me was its investigation of mushroom essences, and I took the opportunity to ask Robert about his innovative work in this realm. He shared with me that mushroom essences address the shadow side of the soul, bringing darkness from the depths of the subconscious to the surface so that we may face and work to resolve these aspects of self.

While Robert may not have been the first herbal practitioner to create and use mushroom essences, he has taken the work further than anyone else to date. Rooted in a lifelong love of plants, an eighteen-year clinical herbal practice, and a fourteen-year in-depth study of mycology and medicinal mushrooms, Robert has devoted himself to the creation and interpretation of the forty-eight mushroom essences treated in this book. Following in the tradition of Dr. Edward Bach, the original creator of flower essences, Robert approaches healing holistically, without disconnecting the body from the soul. Within this paradigm, "disease is in essence the result of conflict between the Soul and the Mind, and will never be eradicated except by spiritual and mental effort."[1] Mushroom essences may make evident the disparities between the personality and the soul that manifest as ailments in the body. They may pose a challenge for us to live true to our dreams and be our highest selves.

When Robert asked me to write this foreword, I asked him to send me a few essences so I could experience them firsthand. After reading partway through the manuscript, I noticed that certain essences and their key issues resonated with me. I wrote to Robert, listing a few that I was drawn to, and I told him that I thought we should have a conversation to choose essences for me to take. He replied that he would send me two unmarked essences of his choice, so that I wouldn't have expectations of their effects, based on the text. I trusted his judgment on this, and soon two bottles arrived in the mail, marked "A" and "B."

Over the course of the next two lunar cycles, I took a few drops of essence before bed each night. In my dream world I had many experiences that reminded me of the changes I needed to make in my waking life to fulfill my greater potential. Things came up in my life that made it difficult to continue without making a proactive change. The two bottles of essences A and B are empty now, but the lessons I learned within my experience of them remain with me. The mushrooms have spoken to me through their vibrational energies imparted into rainwater. All I had to do was listen and be willing to hear what they had to say.

—WILLOUGHBY AREVALO, member of the Radical Mycology
Collective and contributing author of *Radical Mycology*
Vancouver, BC, June 15, 2015

INTRODUCTION

"Keep your thoughts positive because your thoughts become your words.
Keep your words positive because your words become your behavior.
Keep your behavior positive because your behavior becomes your habits.
Keep your habits positive because your habits become your values.
Keep your values positive because your values become your destiny."

—MAHATMA GANDHI

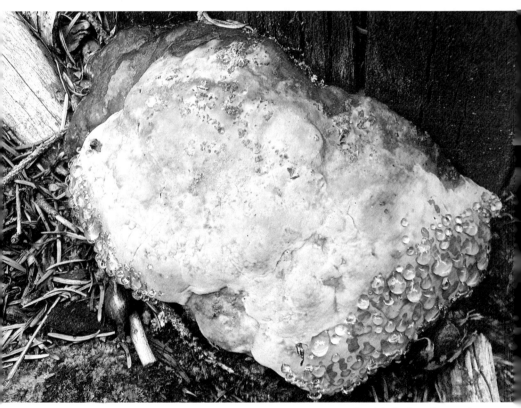

Red-belted conk guttating

Shadow work is humiliating work, but properly so. If you do not "eat" such humiliations with regularity and make friends with all those who reveal to you and convict you of your own denied faults, you will surely remain in the first half of life forever. We never get to the second half of life without major shadowboxing. And I'm sorry to report that it continues until the end of life, the only difference being that you are no longer so surprised by your surprises or so totally humiliated by your humiliations! You come to expect various forms of half-heartedness, deceit, vanity, or illusions from yourself. But now you see through them, which destroys most of their game and power. The important is to learn from your shadow side. Some call this pattern the discovery of the "golden shadow" because it carries so much enlightenment for the soul. The general pattern in story and novel is that heroes learn and grow from encountering their shadow, whereas villains never do.

—RICHARD ROHR

WESTERN CIVILIZATION HAS AN AVERSION TO SHADOW WORK. But why? The answer is that there is hard, honest work involved. As a consequence of this aversion, we now have a modern society run, for the most part, by adolescent males. If this does not frighten you, it should. Many of the major decisions regarding public policy, governance, and our legal system are discussed, written up, and passed into law by immature and juvenile egotists. There are also, however, many mature men and women contributing to our societal well-being and nurturance. You may be one of them.

This book is about helping individuals reconnect with their true authentic self. It is a lifelong process, but one that becomes easier as you increase your soul connection.

WHAT ARE MUSHROOMS?

For a long time mushrooms were believed to be a form of lower plant because they did not produce flowers. It was only in the 1960s that they were given their own kingdom: Fungi. Mushrooms are, in fact, more closely related to humans, and are part of the Opisthokonts. It appears that fungi and animals had a common ancestor sometime after plants went their own direction.

The organism is rarely seen; it grows underground and is connected to herbaceous plants, shrubs, and trees. Over 90 percent of the plants on earth depend on fungi for nutritional support. In exchange for the nutrients and water that the fungi supply through root hairs, the plant delivers life-sustaining sugars. Mushrooms do not contain chlorophyll and, much like humans, cannot produce their own food. It is only the fruiting body that is commonly observed and called a mushroom. This is the reproductive part of fungi.

Lichens are a partnership of algae/cyanobacteria and fungi; this relationship allows them to live in parts of the world where they could not otherwise survive. They are known as extremophiles due to their ability to thrive in extremely hostile environments.

Mushrooms are fascinating. They represent the lymphatic/phlegmatic temperament of our planet. As such, they are constantly feeling and connecting with other aspects of nature. As mentioned, mushrooms and humans are more closely related to each other than to plants. Some four hundred million years ago, a split led to cooperation between mushrooms and plants that allowed both to thrive and evolve on the land. Cyanobacteria (green algae) became the energy producer of plants in the form of chlorophyll, which allowed for sugar production from the energy of the sun. Mushroom mycelia attached to plant roots communicated with plants and offered to exchange water and valuable nutrients in exchange for sugar. Like humans, they cannot manufacture their own food, and they depend on plants for sustenance. Much of the living organism lives underground and produces the sexual organ or fruiting body when it perceives a window of opportunity to successfully reproduce. Communication between the two kingdoms is complex and ever changing, based on climate, environmental conditions, and various stressors, including those caused by humans.

A recent study in Sweden found that the cooperation between plants and mushrooms is less like socialism, or mutual beneficialism, than capitalism. That is, the fungi store up needed materials and water and wait for the best deal from their "sweet daddy" before the exchange takes place. They will hoard and build up reserves waiting for the best deal.

Mushrooms have been sadly neglected by science and often overlooked in terms of their contributions. They are the great decayers of the forest, helping to recycle plant lignans and nutrients to allow for new vegetative growth and healing of scarred landscapes. Mushrooms are the life-blood of the planet, the rhythmic vibration that creates balance and sustainability. They represent order, stability, and health.

WHAT ARE MUSHROOM ESSENCES?

The use of fungi essences is not an entirely new concept, but they have not been very well explored. This could be the result of several factors, including the fungiphobia prevalent throughout much of the English-speaking world.

Mushroom essences are vibrational preparations produced from various parts of the fruiting bodies of the kingdom Fungi. Most essences are made from polypores (spores released from pores), basidiomycetes (gilled mushrooms), and ascomycetes (cup fungi). There are a few lichens, the

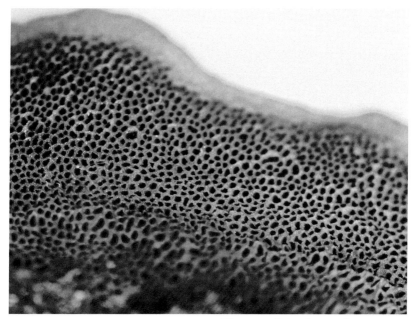

Close-up of cinnabar mushroom pores

unlikely marriage of fungi and algae, and one bryophyte (plant) included in this book.

Mushrooms represent the underbelly or underworld energy of the planet. Unlike flower essences, which are connected to the sun, bringing light into areas of darkness, fungi are lunar, dark, and mysterious.

Like all manner of living beings, they express energetic fields to those willing to observe, listen, and feel. This vibration can in turn be captured and used in clinical and private psychological work. Because no physical substance remains, the mushrooms can do no harm; on the contrary, in the hands of a skilled practitioner, mushroom essences can help peel away the steel bars of long-held emotional and mental imprisonment. By giving the soul permission to express, a practitioner can not only be free to be more authentic, but can assist loved ones, friends, clients, and patients on their own journeys.

Mushroom essences bring awareness to our shadowed side. They represent deep and difficult issues surrounding the "winter of the soul." They represent ancient memory and past-life experience, helping shape our psyche and manner of functioning in the world, not simply in terms of personality, but in regard to the belief systems learned early in life that dictate worldview and focus. Mushrooms represent ancient truths that build character. They support and help us understand the mystery of mythologies and the archetypal hero and heroines of our journey.

The artist Kingsley Gunatillake released an exhibition of giant mushroom abstract paintings in 2006. The Sri Lanka *Sunday Times* wrote insightfully about his allegory of giant mushrooms:

> *Mushrooms tend to sprout in neglected, damp, hidden spots. The dark areas and mushrooms are a metaphor for the apathy in society, which leads to various consequences. The implication is that often people's uncaring and ignorant ways breed "mushrooms"—ill feelings that can ultimately create terrible situations.*
>
> *The mushroom's fragility is also significant because Kingsley believes that crises such as war or crime that emerge due to neglect and misunderstanding can easily be averted or resolved with adequate care and effort.*
>
> *Furthermore, there are several types of mushrooms: some are edible while others are poisonous. Hence the mushroom represents the uncertainty in today's world where one is unsure of one's step, having to be cautious because what lies ahead could be either beneficial or unsafe.[1]*

Václav Hálek, the Mushroom Whisperer, heard mushrooms singing to him starting in 1980. He composed over five thousand mushrooms songs, and in season he added at least one every day during his walks in the woods:

> *Whenever I connect with a mushroom I always have essentially the same two feelings. The first is that the mushroom is pleased that I have noticed it and then it wants to show me what it is and why it is in this world. Then a composition arises. Sometimes I give them a wink when I hear the music.... I've got almost two thousand mushroom types done right now. Some have about twenty compositions, some only one. Let's take the Lepista saeva: it's got*

more than sixty songs, because it keeps on growing even if no other mushroom does.²

Sadly, Hálek passed away in the autumn of 2014.

Mushroom essences are useful for those who wish to address deep personality issues pertaining to emotional or spiritual growth and self-awareness. They are very useful in the context of working with practitioners who understand the challenge associated with change and self-actualization arising from moments of crisis. After all, who but the brave and enlightened would journey on a path of self-discovery that reveals the pitfalls and depths of human suffering and despair?

> *Mature people have somehow picked up the knack of being generous with their sympathies while still taking care of themselves.... The stories of heroes and heroines tell of a journey that takes them from home, across dangerous thresholds, into new, unexplored territories, and then back home with an expanded consciousness. The three phases of this journey—departure, struggle, return—are a metaphor for what happens in us as we evolve from neurotic ego to the spiritual Self. The neurotic ego insists on staying in control and fears the emergence of the Self, which says yes to "what is." The ego's fear of the Self is conditionality fearing unconditionality. Ironically, this is the fear of fearlessness.... All fear is a fear of adulthood, fear of confronting the realities that we did not design or choose....*
>
> *We do not let go of control on our own. Usually, something has to happen that shows us incontrovertibly that we are not in control. From this condition of bankrupt ego, we finally let go. Great losses are thus necessary losses, like the discarded sandbags that lighten a balloon so it can ascend higher.... Loss is a path to gain.³*

In this quotation, David Richo reminds us that we must let go in order to expand and grow. The ego tells us to hold onto what we believe we know and resists any change to the status quo. Elevation to connection with higher self, looking upward, is an important step on the stairway to heaven. Diving down into the belly of the beast is for those seeking stronger connection with soul. Spirit is ascending in a balloon; soul tending is scraping our knees in a rocky cave.

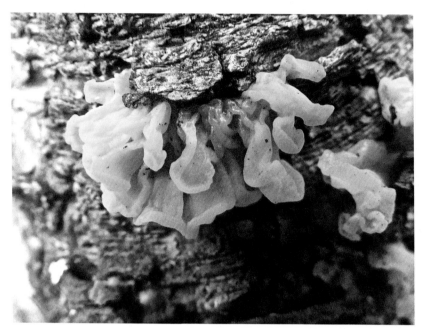

Orange jelly fungus

Martin Ball summarizes these issues well in *Mushroom Wisdom*:

When approached as teachers, however, the mushroom experience, while potentially profoundly joyful, and potentially radically difficult, is primarily work. Learning is work. Understanding our true self is work. Understanding the nature of the mind and our construction of reality is work. But it is work with profound rewards.

To learn from mushrooms takes courage, dedication, and perseverance. They can be brutal teachers, for the truth is often hard to face.

We wrap ourselves in so many illusions and self-generated lies that the mushrooms have to force us out of them to see the truth.... Fear is a powerful force that convinces us to cling to our illusions and our deceptions because even when they make us miserable, at least they make us feel safe and secure.

In many respects, this is a deep pathology in contemporary Western culture—a refusal to look clearly and honestly at the darkness. In Western cultures, the shadow looms very large indeed.[4]

Indeed! Mushroom essences will not do the inner work for us. They are not magic bullets that dissolve our pain, reduce our anger, or assuage our fear. Mushroom essences help create the opportunity for change, the chance to look once more into the abyss of unresolved and buried angst, and create an abundance of excitation in being alive. They stir up the psyche, shake the shadows, and reveal old patterns that prevent us from connection with soul. Mushroom essences represent the roots of various archetypal negative emotions, and help nurture and guide us to a greater understanding of our formative patterns.

Imagine an ancient tree. The branches and leaves and flowers represent the splendor and creative joy of expression. The trunk represents long-standing growth, the annual rings of expansion and contraction. The roots sink deeply into the earth, creating stability. And the underworld mycelia of mushrooms nurture and feed. They embody the true nature of character and soul—our roots and root chakras, if you will.

Flower essence practitioners will find mushroom essences create synergistic potential. Clare Harvey puts it well:

> Mushroom essences are perfectly suited to match or complement flower essences. In these combinations, flower essences act on the emotional body, while mushroom essences carry these changes to the physical level, integrating the energy absorbed into the cells. As mushroom essences can have a very strong effect they need to be tested before use. They enter deep into our subconscious revealing deeply buried issues. Timing is all important when taking mushroom essences; the individual personality needs to be mature enough to cope with confrontation of deep issues and be able to process the information that is released.[5]

CHAPTER 1

THE JOURNEY
OF DISCOVERING
MUSHROOM ESSENCES

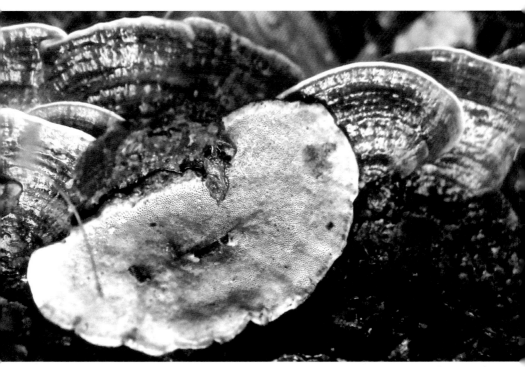

Rosy conk

A number of techniques were utilized in the development of these mushroom essences. I had the good fortune to have a clinical practice as a professional herbalist for eighteen years, and I utilized flower and mushroom essences while working with clients.

In some cases, the mushrooms just "spoke" to me, similar to the manner in which our beloved Czech composer heard music. I respect that some individuals will have trouble with this concept, but I remember talking to several shamans in Peru in the early 1980s, asking them how they knew which plant was good for a specific condition. They looked at me with puzzlement, and then replied simply that the plant told them.

In other cases I utilized the doctrine of signature as a gateway to revealing the emotional and spiritual properties of various fungi. I would be drawn to the shape, color, or even the energetics of the environment in which they appeared. And the journey began.

Julia Graves contributes to this discussion:

> *The doctrine of signatures is really a poetic language describing a multidimensional reality in which different facets of signature are simultaneously true, and in which the interplay of the countless elements cannot be exhaustively and finally interpreted. Since it is the human mind that gives meaning to nature, naturally the signatures and their categories shift from one cultural context to another, one adding to the other without contradiction but rather contributing another piece to the larger picture.... The art of interpreting poetry means that there is never just one meaning, and that one can never find all the meanings.*[1]

Matthew Wood suggests, "The doctrine of signatures operates through at least two different subjective faculties, the intuition and the imagination."[2] Intuition is the ability to see patterns in the world, and imagination is the ability to see images.

I took my work one step further. After preparing different mushroom essences, I ingested them during dream time and journeys, and noted and recorded my impressions. I taught herbal and mushroom medicine for ten years at a university and even longer at Northern

Star College, co-owned by my wife and other amazing practitioners. I was easily able to encourage student experimentation with various essences, tracking and following their individual journeys. There is no end to this work. If you experience a breakthrough, or an impression, from any of the mushroom essences, feel free to share it with me for inclusion in a revised edition.

CAUTION: There is no physical matter in any of these essences. Individuals may experience impressions based on their own subjective interpretations. The case studies with each of the mushroom essences are examples to help the reader understand the possible use for various emotional responses on the journey to integration with soul. No two individuals will experience the essences in the same way, nor should there be any such expectation.

THE FUNGAL-CHEMICAL PROCESS

Kingdom Fungi is more than a metaphor for mystery, fear, and the unknown. Similar to *Homo sapiens* searching for the philosopher's stone, mushrooms and lichens recycle, transmute, and transform. Harmful matter is turned into something of value. Many alchemists use a seven-step process when referring to the cycle of changing lead to gold—or using human characteristics, changing something flawed into something precious. For all humans, there comes a time for transformation. Like humans, mushrooms exhibit the various stages of growth necessary for connection to soul. Here are the seven steps.

Calcination

The first step of alchemy is calcination, where a substance is burned until only ash remains. Thunder and lightning are present, promoting visitation with flashes of intuition and imagination. It was believed in ancient times and throughout various cultures that mushrooms would appear after thunder and lightning. In Japan, oak logs were pounded with hammers to simulate thunderous vibrations to increase the fruiting yield of shiitake mushrooms.

Calcination represents the destruction of ego and attachment to material goods. It is working with fire to ignite a passion in our souls. Fire morel mushrooms are such an example, rising like the phoenix from the ashes of a previous year's forest fire.

Dissolution

Dissolution soon follows and relates to the ash dissolving in fluid, including water and rain. Minerals are dissolved to an ionic phase by the mycorrhizal networks. It is a step of cultivating detachment, but also related to creativity and the catalyst for sexuality. This is an unconscious process, where buried material is revealed and life begins to flow. It is the stage of creative acts and release of prejudice. Fear of institutions and established hierarchy is dissolved at this stage. The split gill mushroom, for example, exhibits over twenty-eight thousand various sexual expressions.

This is where the connection between soul and sex is manifest, at the root chakra. Minerals are dissolved to an ionic phase and exchanged via root hairs of neighboring plants for the sweet molecules of life. The exchange of nutrients with plants is not altruistic, but is a bargaining between mutually benefiting organisms.

Separation

The third stage, separation, is about coming apart. For fungi, this represents gaining new territory and advancing into unknown space. Arguably the largest organism on earth, the honey mushroom's massive size is mainly underground. It thrives with awareness of time but retains a sense of boundary.

This is the stage of retaining what is useful and discarding the rest. The shadow is reexamined, and self-inflicted wounds are released so that our true nature can come through. Adversity sharpens the process of separation and encourages movement from under to upper. As above, so below.

Conjunction

The fourth stage is conjunction, where opposite elements reunite. Separation is two minus one. The synergy created is one plus one equals three. Lichens are a perfect example of fungi and algae coming together to create what each could not achieve on their own. They represent the respiration system and lungs of the planet. Territory is transmuted to integrity. The process translates intention that is hard-won and persistent. It is the union of male and female, a unified state of consciousness.

Fungi require protein—the building blocks of life—and they lasso nematodes and paralyze springtails for nourishment. The growing mycelial fibers transmit intelligence and contain the rhythm or heartbeat of our planet. This process illustrates the complex and fragile, strong and united qualities of the kingdom. Conjunction develops empathy, compassion, and a reuniting of intention.

Fermentation

The fifth stage, although often the most difficult for humans, seems natural for fungi. Fermentation means a substance will not change unless it is left alone in the dark. While most humans tend to fight this very uncomfortable state of depression and depth, fungi, born of the dark, appear to thrive.

Unlike the traditional stage of alchemy where the goal is to transform lead into gold, the fung-alchemical process turns lead, mercury, and other heavy metals and petroleum hydrocarbon toxins into the basic elements of carbon, nitrogen, hydrogen, and oxygen. Fungi translocate metals of the periodic table into the building blocks of life.

Humans, at this stage of transition, experience the dark night of the soul. We require an adjustment of will, as in, "Thy will be done." Individuals attracted to the healing arts may experience a personal health challenge. The ego of "I am the healer" is reexamined and replaced with empathy and compassion.

There are two sides of soul and spirit, between matter and mind. Fermentation is a discovery of the living inspiration that did not previously exist. Carl Jung suggested only the wounded physician heals and can only heal others to the extent they have healed themselves.[1] This is true.

Appreciation for silence, stillness, and changing deeply from within can help make this process more tolerable to the human ego, which feels safer in conditions of light and expansion. The lunar stage of growth instead requires depth, dark, and acceptance. It has its own rhythm and will be set back by intolerance and impatience.

Unique vibrational essences prepared from fungi and lichens address many of the negative moods and emotions, as well as full moon and lunar traumas of the psyche. They help address archetypal human fragility and support connection with soul.

Sublimation

The sixth stage is sublimation, or distillation, where the essence rises to the top. Symptoms associated with this stage are confusion, hyperactivity, and feeling out of control. Fruiting bodies of *Psilocybe* and related species represent conscious awareness and magical intuition. This is the culmination of the five previous steps, and our collective source of wisdom and change.

Magic and mushrooms impact others around them, with shared visions and dreams. Sublimation brings out the creativity and connects us with soul, instead of ego. Distillation brings introspection that raises the psyche to its highest possible level.

Rituals are introduced to help aid concentration and intention. Various fungi contain volatile oils, produced by distillation, that represent essence. These help to soothe the skin and protect this valuable layer that creates the sense of self and attracts like-minded individuals. It initiates mastery of the natural laws of cause and effect.

Coagulation

The final stage is coagulation or illumination, the forming of the philosopher's stone. This solid landscape is a place of sacred magic and surrender. Various fungi, especially members of the *Mycena* and *Panellus* genera, exhibit myco-luminescence, representing enlightenment. They shine because they can. They express because they know.

A new sense of confidence emerges, creating awareness throughout many levels of reality. It is attunement with the higher self, and a living

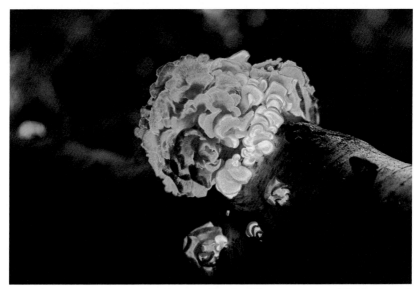
Luminescent *Panellus* (photo courtesy of Keith Garrett)

wisdom of intention and widened perception. This is the resurrection of the soul: the complete connection of inner and outer self. As within, so without. Existence is experienced on all levels at the same time. Jung calls this the process of individuation. Finally, the fung-alchemical process is complete.

HOW TO PREPARE AND USE MUSHROOM ESSENCES

Mushroom essences are produced from the fruiting bodies, burned ash, spores, guttation (sweat), mycelia, hydrosols, deliquescing ink, or parts thereof, making them quite different from flower essences. For example, crab apple is one of Bach's original flower essences and is produced from new flowers layered on spring water in sunlight. The equivalent of a fruiting body is the crab apple itself, a very different vibration.

This has much do with the organism and how it reproduces. That is, the underground fungus may be extremely ancient, and patiently waits for the right conditions to reproduce and send its spores to their next destiny. Tree polypores may be either annuals or perennials.

Like flowers, some mushrooms depend on insects for the dispersal of spores and increase their ability to move around the planet. Some spores are so light they can travel in the jet stream hundreds of miles high and descend on different continents.

Mushrooms can accumulate heavy metals, so it is critical to harvest and prepare essences in unpolluted environments. The myco-accumulation of toxins, originating from industrial sites, commercial agriculture, highways, and cities, is to be avoided. The harvesting of mushrooms for essence production should be conducted in pristine and ecologically sound environments.

Most mushroom essences are produced during a full moon, sometimes during the waning or waxing period of the lunar cycle, or over a full twenty-eight-day and night cycle. The lichens are a combination of solar and lunar influence. In some cases, where indicated, a 10 percent portion of colloidal silver is added to twenty-eight lunar cycle preparations to increase energetics and help ensure preservation. The relationship between the metal silver and the moon is ancient. Silver coins from ancient Greece were known as tears of the moon or Owls of Athens. Why the moon? Since ancient times, the various phases of the lunar cycle have given a sense of measurement and time. The moon phases relate to phases in life. In *The Myth of the Goddess* Anne Baring and Jules Cashford write:

> *It is possible that an ability to think abstractly developed from an understanding of the moon's phases as four instead of three. To the three visible phases—the waxing, the full, and the waning—was added the fourth phase, the three days' darkness where the moon cannot be seen and can only be imagined. The fourth, invisible phase may have been understood as the invisible dimension where new life is gestated and from which the old moon is reborn as the new moon.[1]*

In order to be reborn, a part of self must die. Soul work is such a process and may be assisted by mushroom essences. They continue:

> *The skills they developed in observing the phases of the moon and the circular movement of the stars, the stories they told to accompany these rituals, all expressed the specifically human instinct to*

recognize analogies between different orders and dimensions of life. It must have been this power to think analogically that enabled them to perceive the relationship between a heavenly order, symbolized by the moon, and the earthly order they saw around them.

The moon was undoubtedly the central image of the sacred to these early people because, in its dual rhythm of constancy and change, it provided not only a point of orientation from which differences could be measured, patterns conceived and connections made, but also, in its perpetual return to its own beginnings, it unified what had apparently been broken asunder.[2]

Our moon sign is the feminine aspect of an individual. As a mushroom essence is to a flower essence, toward a more subconscious lesser-known element, the astrological moon sign is toward our sun sign. This mysterious, subconscious river holds great motivation and internal energy. Solar energy relates to spirit, lunar energy is soul work. The former connects us to our heavenly sphere, but the latter relates to underworld metamorphosis.

To determine the placement of your moon sign, you will need your birth date and approximate time and place. You can easily find this by using a number of websites, or asking your local astrologer. Learning about your moon sign will provide illumination about your emotional and subconscious nature. Creating the mushroom essence under a particular moon sign may unify or enhance the traits associated with that sign.

Mushroom essences reflect the duality of the psyche, the shattering and bringing together of fragile parts of the soul into a united whole: from disconnection, separation, and fragmentation to cohesion, transformation, and wholeness.

A pure crystal bowl or goblet made of real crystal is filled with pure rainwater. When not available, spring water may be substituted, but do not use tap water, as it is toxic, or distilled water, as it is inert. Then, the fruiting body, spores, or "ink" are placed on the surface of the water. It is important to avoid direct handling, so use a pair of wooden, not metal, chopsticks to transfer the fruiting body to the crystal bowl. Use a ceramic knife to prepare certain mushrooms. Mushroom and lichen essences are prepared in a specific manner, and directions for each are found at the end of every chapter.

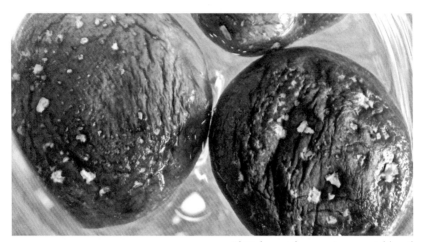

Shiitake mushrooms in a crystal bowl

Various lunar phases will subtly influence the energy of a mushroom essence. In most cases, a lunar influence of at least four hours is desired. In some cases, it is difficult to find and prepare an essence exactly on the full moon. In this case, the preparation during the waxing or waning phases will influence the essence energetics slightly. The waxing moon phase, building toward full, is more restorative and restful, gathering strength, storing energy, absorbing, building up, taking in, planning, and breathing in. A waning moon phase is the opposite; it detoxifies, removes, breathes out, hardens, and dries the emotions, and it is related to action and expenditure of energy. The differences are subtle, in many cases, but where indicated for particular essences, will add additional energetic influence.

The strained water is added to additional rain or spring water, boiled, cooled, and then added to 80 percent brandy or moonshine. This creates the so-called mother stock. Next is succusion, a technique used at both the mother-stock and dosage-bottle stages of preparation. In homeopathy, succusion is a means of potentiating the essence. The bottle is gently agitated by striking it into the palm of the hand one hundred times. The term *succusion* is from the German *schütteln*.

The next step is to take four drops of this preparation and add it to a 30 percent brandy and water mixture in an amber glass dropper bottle. This is known as the stock bottle and is the form in which mushroom essences are commercially available. This is also succussed.

Using Mushroom Essences

Taking a single or combination of mushroom essences for a full lunar cycle is indicated in most cases. They may be started at any phase of the lunar cycle. No more than three mushroom essences should be combined and taken together at one time. Four drops of the stock remedy are added to a 30-milliliter dropper bottle with equal parts water and brandy or moonshine. This is succussed, and then just four drops are taken before bedtime for twenty-eight days.

CHAPTER 2

THE MUSHROOM ESSENCES

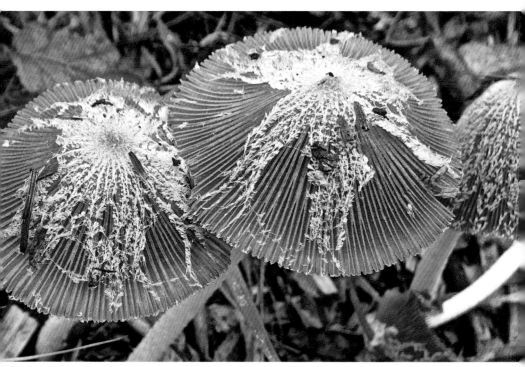

Harefoot mushroom (*Coprinopsis lagopus*)

VARNISH CONK

(Ganoderma tsugae)

INDICATIONS: conformity, self-love, timelessness, money, transformation, authenticity, true path, PTSD

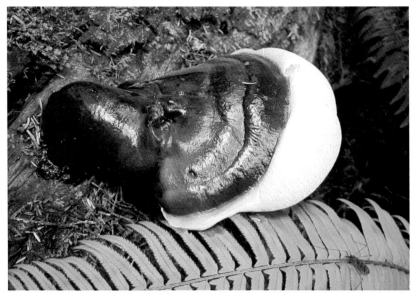

Varnish conk (*Ganoderma tsugae* Murrill)

Two roads diverged in a wood, and I, I took the one less traveled by, and that has made all the difference.
—ROBERT FROST

The opposite of courage in our society is not cowardice, it is conformity.
—ROLLO MAY

In America, through pressure of conformity, there is freedom of choice, but nothing to choose from.
—PETER USTINOV

Ganoderma is from the Latin *gan,* for "shiny," and *derm,* meaning "skin." *Tsugae* refers to its favorite host, hemlock spruce, although it also loves western larch and Douglas fir. It is a very close cousin to, and in fact may be part of, the larger *Ganoderma lucidum* complex.

Varnish conk exhibits a reddish-orange-brown and white surface. Brown and red represent the root chakra, our center of survival and basic flight-and-fright level of feeling grounded. Red and brown represent birth and rebirth, as well as blood, bone, and muscle tissue. Orange represents the second or sexual chakra, and white is associated with the crown chakra at the top of the head. Energy moves from our root to our crown chakra when unimpeded by blockages. Red represents blood as well as heat and inflammation in body tissue. White represents the healing of bones. There is often a small golden band between the white and orange-brown areas, suggestive of heart and spirituality.

The shape of this annual polypore varies, but it is generally lung-like, or sometimes in the form of a kidney. The smell is damp and earthy, with a bittersweet odor that becomes more obvious with a small bite into the young, fresh fruiting body.

Essence Description

Varnish conk mushroom essence is associated with issues of death, transformation, and immortality. In ancient times, it was believed to rouse the dead. Raven-like birds placed the fungus on the faces of dead men, who immediately sat up and were restored to life. In China, the raven is a solar bird associated with good omens and fetching of light into the world,[1] according to Frans Vermeulen.

Varnish conk mushroom essence is also associated with finding our true path in life. It is easy to fall into patterns of pleasing others, particularly our families, and then later, our teachers and employers. Our seat of passion will boil and bubble unless listened to and acted upon.

The striving for financial success may at times compromise our deep-seated basic philosophy of life. All around us will be people encouraging the accumulation of material goods as *the* path to happiness. This may be the result of an early connection with poverty, or a lineage of parents and grandparents who never felt enough physical or fiscal support. But true contentment is found in the root chakra, where on a daily basis there is a feeling of safety and security associated with being ourselves. Without a secure foundation, we cannot reach for the sky and fully explore the scope of universal understanding and fulfillment.

The new edition of the *Diagnostic and Statistical Manual of Mental Disorders* (DSM-5) defines a new mental illness called oppositional defiant disorder, or ODD. This is an "ongoing pattern of disobedient, hostile, and defiant behavior" including symptoms such as questioning authority, negativity, defiance, argumentativeness, and being easily annoyed. Other new mental illnesses defined by the DSM-5 include arrogance, narcissism, above-average creativity, cynicism, and antisocial behavior. There are a large variety of pharmaceutical treatments available. Of course there are—the manual is published by the American Psychiatric Association. An article in the *Washington Post* noted that if Mozart were born today, he would be diagnosed with attention deficit disorder and "medicated into barren normality."[2]

Varnish conk mushroom essence may help individuals who are free-thinking and nonconformist, conditions now considered mental illnesses. Finding our true self is a soul journey that requires support, regardless of our individual personality traits. To become authentic requires becoming clear with our true desires, values, and emotions. Group consciousness can easily sway those individuals feeling insecure or unsure of themselves. In time, authenticity and integrity become the basis of a new path of living. To secure this authenticity, we must express it verbally. This involves learning the difference between various levels of shallow and deep loyalty.

To become one with nature and flow with the river is to be open to new adventures, new friendships, and expanded concepts of self-love. This does not mean putting our own interests above those of others, but rather feeling in touch with the beauty of the inner self.

Varnish conk mushroom essence helps us explore deep-seated belief systems formed before conscious thought. Many of our early childhood learnings and perceptions of the world were filtered through the eyes of our parents, with their unspoken bias and prejudice. Core issues of self often require the individual steps of recognition, discernment, and continuing the process.

This mushroom essence works slowly and creates a sense of time-lessness. It transfers the linear into the expansive, and transforms perceptions of death and dying into expansion, connection, and awareness of soul. In order to grow, parts of self must die and be reborn.

It should be used in small doses, by individuals who have suffered first chakra injury, including post–traumatic stress disorder, childhood abandonment, and psychic wounds related to survival issues around food, air, water, and shelter.

Society pushes us toward conformity, not soul purpose. This mushroom essence helps bring awareness to this issue. In cases of early traumas associated with umbilical cords wrapped around the neck at birth, near drownings, fetal starvation, and so on, take the drops as suggested, but note the dream states that appear. If bringing forth awareness of repressed memory is too frightening, stop for a period of time, or go more slowly. It is an ideal adjunct remedy for Rebirthing Therapy.

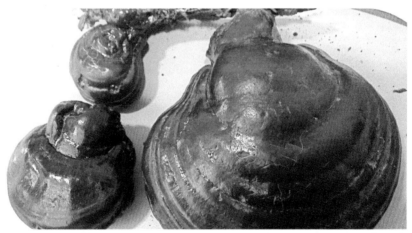

Varnish conk

PREPARATION AND USE: The essence is produced from slices of the whole fresh fruiting body, on the surface of fresh rainwater, in a crystal bowl under lunar influence. To enhance individualistic tendencies, prepare the mushroom essence with the moon in Aquarius. To strengthen regenerative aspects, make the essence while the moon is in Scorpio.

CASE STUDY: Stewart was a new client, forty-eight years old, married for twenty-eight years, with two children. He was a chartered accountant, in his own words "sick and tired" of work. He wanted a career change but was fearful of financial security issues and responsibilities. "It seems that money is running my life."

I suggested varnish conk mushroom essence drops may be helpful taken as indicated for a full lunar cycle. Before the lunar cycle was complete, he quit his job and took his wife and children on a second honeymoon. Upon their return home, he began a new career in landscape architecture.

CASE STUDY: Diane was a twenty-three-year-old single postal clerk. She came to my clinic suffering from asthma and painful menstrual periods. She was diagnosed at age six with asthma and had been on increasingly strong medications for a number of years. She noted a caduceus symbol on my office wall and commented, "I hate snakes." I noted her blouse was loose at the neck and asked if she minded tight collars. I recommended homeopathic *Lachesis,* a snake venom remedy, and varnish conk mushroom essence for one lunar cycle. I also suggested she keep a dream journal. She returned with large smile on her face. Both her menstrual cycle and respiratory issues were significantly improved.

We went over her dream journal together, and I noted one entry of interest. She was walking a large dog around a lake, and it turned into a wolf. The leash was torn from her hands and became a large chain that was wrapped around her neck. The next moment, she was being dragged into the lake and pulled underwater. She woke up, gasping for air and feeling pain in her throat. At that moment, she recalled her mother telling her she had almost died at birth, with the cord wrapped around her neck.

I recommended she make an appointment with a colleague who practiced Rebirthing Therapy. She made excellent progress.

ARTIST'S CONK

(Ganoderma applanatum)

INDICATIONS: despair, empathy, nature versus nurture, nature deficit disorder

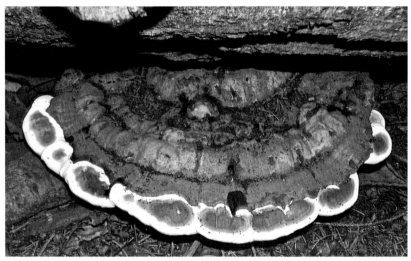

Artist's conk (*Ganoderma applanatum* [Persoon] Patouillard)

Nature's patterns sometimes reflect two intertwined features:
fundamental physical laws and environmental influences.
It's nature's version of nature versus nurture.

—BRIAN GREENE

Nature is often obscure, but she is not, like man, deceitful. The dream
itself wants nothing: it is a self-evident content, a plain natural fact.

—CARL JUNG

Artist's conk is generally less shiny than its cousin *G. tsugae*. The species name *applanatum* is from the Latin, meaning "flattened." The common name refers to use of the white spore-bearing lower surface by artists for sketching and painting. Art is, of course, a true expression of soul.

There is considerable variation with artist's conk, but in general, the surface is more brown than red, with new white growth appearing annually on the outside perimeter. The color brown is associated with earthiness. It relates to an acceptance of the impermanence of life.

The annual white regrowth represents the central nervous system, or a sense of inner peace and oneness. White is the color of the crown chakra and affects all other chakras. Each year, the perennial polypore creates new growth and can, over time, become very large and expansive. Similar to humans, they can live up to one hundred years or more in old growth forests. During the prime time of summer, a large mushroom will produce up to twenty-one million spores a minute.

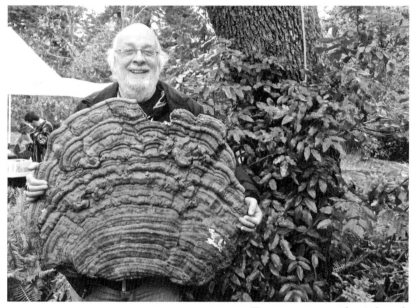

Twenty-two-pound artist's conk

Essence Description

Artist's conk mushroom essence helps us develop a more supportive nature. To many women, especially mothers, this may simply be second nature. But to many men, this may be a place of trepidation and fear.

Artist's conk represents the archetypal conflict of nurture and nature. The mushroom essence assists those who value self-reliance as a virtue and helps us take a second look at how we can assist others on their own personal journey to soul connection.

The mushroom essence helps us remember how a few individuals were, at some point, important early teachers on our path to maturity. Paying it forward is the message of this mushroom essence.

Artist's conk helps us find an ideal balance of receptive femininity and assertive masculinity. This is a different path for everyone. Early in life, many young boys are taught to not cry, in the belief that this attitude will toughen and strengthen them on their road to becoming real men. Evidence suggests the contrary, and for adult men, the inability to emote, show empathy, and console one another becomes more difficult. The artist's conk may be combined with red-belted conk mushroom essence for this particular issue.

The shadow side addressed by this mushroom essence is the pervasive belief that nature is to be conquered and overcome. This essence helps us understand that people are part of nature, and what harms nature is detrimental to all living beings, including humans. Preteen and teenage children would greatly benefit from a deeper connection with nature as a pathway to soul, but unfortunately many adults and teachers are themselves unaware of the path.

One example is the forestry worker or logger who earns an income cutting down old-growth forests. This person may be fully committed to providing for his family but has lost touch with the interconnected web of life. To his eyes, the trees look like dollar signs. In fact, many individuals working in forestry, both commercial and governmental, see mushrooms as a wood-rot organism, killing *their* trees that are harvested for profit. Nature versus nurture: this inner conflict can lead to crises of conscience and the so-called "dark night of the soul." In reality, sustainable harvest is both attainable and practiced in many parts of our planet.

Artist's conk mushroom essence helps us understand that the world's forests are everyone's legacy. It helps bring to awareness the realization that our forests are the lungs of the planet, and they are grieving their destruction. Wilderness is not wild; it is in perfect balance. The human is the only species that has great difficulty in understanding that it is part of nature, not the top of the pyramid.

This essence is useful for teachers and mentors helping shape the minds of today's students. More than ever, young people are starved for connection with nature. As Richard Louv writes, "The children and nature movement is fueled by this fundamental idea: the child in nature is an endangered species, and the health of children and the health of the earth are inseparable."[3]

Artist's conk mushroom essence may help alleviate, or put into proper perspective, the tortured feelings of despair suffered by many ecologists and environmentalists. For sensitive individuals, each new wound on Gaia opens a response of pain and suffering. To witness destructive clear-cutting in the boreal or Amazon forests can be devastating to the fragile psyche. Artist's conk helps us align with our true nature and relationship as part of the larger soul purpose.

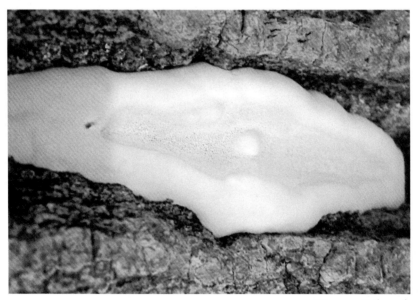

Young artist's conk

PREPARATION: The essence of artist's conk is prepared with a layer of spores covering rainwater in a crystal bowl for one lunar night, if the sky is mainly clear. Overnight, the spores will slowly sink to the bottom of the bowl. Remove the top half of the water with a pipette and combine with brandy.

Under Taurus, the influence is more toward nature, and under Cancer, more toward nurturance.

CASE STUDY: Jason was a single twenty-seven-year-old oil-rig worker living in a northern camp with eight thousand other employees. He suffered from daily headaches, joint pain, partial limb paralysis, dizziness, and poor concentration. He despaired over the environmental impact associated with his job, but he said he needed the money. I suggested he try artist's conk mushroom essence, as directed, for an entire lunar cycle.

On his next visit, he reported a mild cessation of many symptoms, including headaches and dizziness. His concentration was greatly improved, and he had stopped drinking alcohol. Another lunar cycle of mushroom essence was suggested, and he agreed. But he did not book another appointment.

One year later, he came to see me. He said that halfway through the second cycle, he quit his job and moved back to the family farm. He had taken over the farm from his elderly father and had begun the process of converting the land to organic certification. He looked incredibly strong, healthy, and happy.

COMB TOOTH
(Hericium coralloides)

INDICATIONS: cellular memory, Alzheimer's disease, concentration

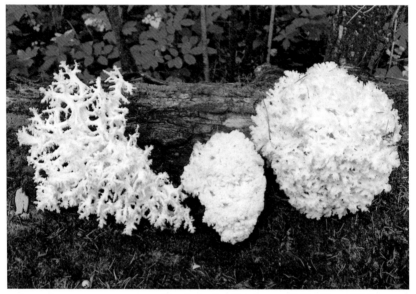

Comb tooth (*Hericium coralloides* [Scopoli] Persoon)

No matter how closely you examine the water, glucose,
and electrolyte salts in the human brain, you can't find
the point where these molecules became conscious.
—DEEPAK CHOPRA

In the practical use of our intellect, forgetting
is as important as remembering.
—WILLIAM JAMES

Looking for consciousness in the brain is like
looking inside a radio for the announcer.
—NASSIM HARAMEIN

Hericium or comb tooth is a pure white, branched mushroom. Its intricate growth suggests to the imagination a series of brain neurons. In fact, recent research indicates that water-soluble compounds from this mushroom cross the blood-brain barrier and promote brain neuron growth. This suggests the need for more research into a natural approach for senile dementia, multiple sclerosis, and Alzheimer's disease.

The color white represents purity, cleanliness, and light, and is associated with the crown chakra on top of the body.

The fruiting bodies express themselves in a variety of ways, mainly around the concept of concentration and expansion. Note in the photo the three examples of fruiting bodies growing together on the same tree. They vary in growth from a concentrated brain lobe–like concentration to an expansive filamentary radiance. The dangling expressions are reminiscent of nerve endings and tendrils of tenderness.

Ralph Twentyman noted the connection between nerves and fungi:

> *Throughout our bodies, these [nerve] fibers ramify, and it is estimated that if all these fibers were joined together into a single thread, they would go around the world twelve times. The nerve man then is a web of nerve fibers, and even the apparently solid nervous organs, the spinal cord and brain, are composed of these fibers. One-dimensionality dominates; there are no leaves, no real membranes or surfaces. We are forcibly reminded of the world of fungi, whose structure, even of the mushroom, is composed of one-dimensional fibers, at the most matted together. Fungi are mycelial threads, and at the ends they may turn into spores or dust. The fungi, too, live parasitically off decaying vegetable and animal matter, reducing them also to dust.[4]*

In Western society, the brain often overrules the heart. We are taught that the left side of the brain is related to intellect, decision-making, precision, and linear thinking, and the right side is more creative, spatial, artistic, and expansive. The enteric brain, which is rich in hormone-producing tissue, is found in the intestine and produces the majority of dopamine, serotonin, and noradrenaline in our body.

Brain health relates to short- and long-term memory and is considered the conductor of the orchestra. Nothing could be farther from the truth. The majority of life trauma is stored in muscle tissues throughout the body and held there until released. Deep tissue release, Rolfing, and other bodywork can help release stored patterns of negativity.

Our soul remembers every lifetime but does not share this information with conscious memory.

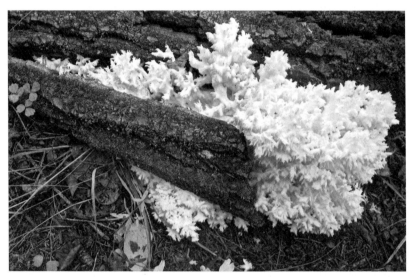

Young comb tooth

Essence Description

Comb tooth mushroom essence assists us by awakening cellular memory, which is then "remembered" in dream-time or by disturbances in the connective tissue of the body. Past-life memories and experiences may come to the surface, helping release old patterns of holding on, or bringing awareness to painful and unpleasant trauma.

The essence may be thought of as a reconnection to the various soul experiences that brought us to this time and place. From every learning experience, there is a memory to assist the process of our journey to awareness and enlightenment. Memory of our descent into the other world helps us attune to our individuation. Attention to tissue discomfort will assist the mental, emotional, and spiritual process of integration, information, intuition, and imagination.

Jung noted, "All the works of man have their origin in creative fantasy. What right have we then to depreciate imagination?"[5] Jung spoke of racial memories as feelings and ideas inherited from our ancestors as part of the collective unconscious. Mice trained to fear a specific smell will pass on this aversion to later generations never exposed to it or trained to fear it. The researchers of this study concluded: "The experiences of a parent, even before conceiving, markedly influence both the structure and function in the nervous system of subsequent generations."[6] This suggests epigenetic influence.

Neurons throughout the body respond to stimuli of all types by growth and expansion. Repetition of old patterns will stunt growth and reinforce old stereotypes of repressed memory. Individuals feel stuck or unable to move on.

Comb tooth essence helps reset our tingle factor. When new awareness combines with deep-seated traditional memory, it creates opportunity for blissful moment-to-moment living. It helps us feel alive and be more appreciative of loving partners, friends, and community.

PREPARATION: Comb tooth essence is prepared by covering rainwater with fresh fruiting bodies in a crystal bowl during a moon influenced by Aries or Gemini.

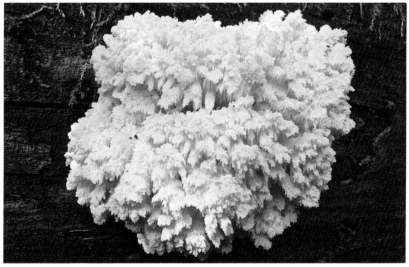

Mature comb tooth

CASE STUDY: Stacey was a thirty-three-year-old single woman, working as a retail clerk. She came to see me suffering from "brain fog," poor concentration, and in her words, just "feeling bland." Her dreams were seldom remembered, and those few were black-and-white. She began taking the mushroom essence for a lunar cycle and later reported that by day ten, she was dreaming in Technicolor.

I asked her to keep a dream journal. One night, she saw herself as a seven-year-old girl suffering from epilepsy. She recalled that for eight years she was given daily doses of Dilantin to prevent seizures, based on a single isolated event. Comb tooth mushroom essence was repeated for a second lunar cycle, with significant improvement in her memory and vitality. I added bearberry flower essence, from the Prairie Deva line, to assist with movement of energy up the spine.

She began to release mental and physical numbness and started coming back into her body. She said, "It feels like a mild shiver moving from my lower back to the top of my head. I was scared at first, but now I kind of like it."

RED-BELTED CONK
(Fomitopsis pinicola)

INDICATIONS: deception, denial, arthritis, discernment, flexibility, responsibility, rigidity

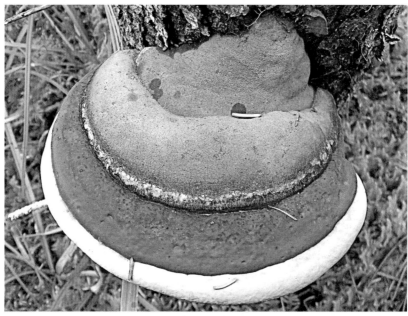

Red-belted conk (*Fomitopsis pinicola* [Swartz] Karsten)

Tears are the summer showers to the soul.

—ALFRED AUSTIN

If it's never our fault, we can't take responsibility for it. If we can't take responsibility for it, we'll always be its victim.

—RICHARD BACH

Most men cry better than they speak.

—HENRY DAVID THOREAU

Fomitopsis means "fomes-like," and *pinicola* means "pine-loving," suggesting it prefers the company of members of the pine family. This includes fir, spruce, larch, hemlock, and, of course, pine. But I have seen it equally at home on deciduous trees such as poplar, birch, alder, and maple. Red-belted conk comes in nearly every color of the rainbow except green, ranging from red to orange, yellow, blue, violet, and white.

The energy is warm and moist, helping relieve painful arthritis and various cold conditions of rheumatism and other muscular and skeletal inflammation. Most noticeable is the tendency for the fruiting bodies to guttate, or sweat. The chemical analysis of this secretion is not yet complete, and it may lead to some interesting compounds. Essential oils and hydrosols contain unique compounds not found in plant material but stored in secretory glands. These tears are the key signature.

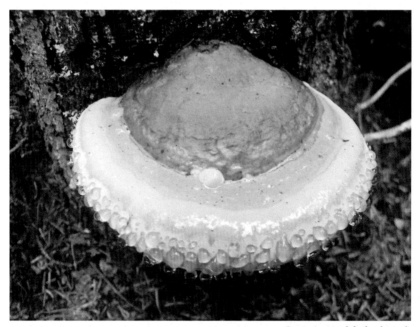

Guttating red-belted conk

Essence Description

Red-belted conk mushroom essence is associated with responsibility and flexibility, which are related in a number of ways. Responsibility is the ability to respond, to take action whenever necessary. To flex may mean to bend or adjust to external or internal pressure, or it may suggest a show of strength, such as demonstrating our skills. Both traits are useful throughout various growing phases of our lives. Being responsible for our actions is the cornerstone of a life filled with integrity. The many mistakes that we learn from give us the strength to grow and mature.

Unfortunately, many children learn a better survival technique, involving deception, deflection, denial, and playing victim. This pattern, if repeated with success, can lead to social and criminal behavior and the destruction of interpersonal relationships.

Men and women possess tear glands that are structurally different. Before puberty, girls and boys cry about the same amount, but by age eighteen, young women tear more readily. Tears contain thirty times the concentration of manganese found in our blood. Manganese is considered by many health practitioners to be our "love" element. This trace mineral is particularly useful to the pituitary. Research has found emotional tears of sadness and grief contain more toxins than tears of joy.

Red-belted conk essence helps us rediscover, own, and release our unproductive patterns. The ability to respond suggests we have the emotional capacity and courage to stand up for what we believe. Crocodile tears, used for manipulative purposes, will dry up.

Flexibility is the virtue of discernment: knowing when to move forward and when to retreat. It could be said it involves knowing when and where to pick our battles. It does not mean we choose to move around an issue due to lack of bravery, but rather because we have more important things to accomplish. The opposite of flexibility is rigidity, suggestive of hanging on to belief systems, creating less space and fewer options in life. Given space, soul has room to relax, expand, and grow. Red-belted conk helps us give ourselves permission to pursue opportunities for soul growth.

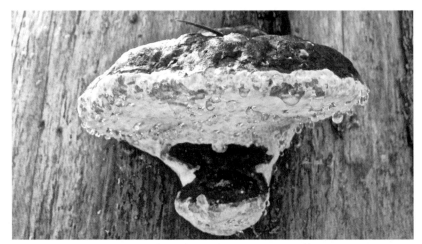

Guttating red-belted conk

PREPARATION: This mushroom mother essence is prepared directly from the guttation or sweat formed on various red-belted conks, and combined in a one-to-one ratio with brandy. Use a dropper to collect the guttation and then add brandy at the first opportunity. Lunar influence and the astrological influence of Capricorn enhances this essence.

CASE STUDY: Karen was a sixty-two-year-old recently divorced woman with two grown children. She suffered for the previous eighteen years from rheumatoid arthritis. She was deeply religious and a member of Al-Anon, as her former spouse was an alcoholic. I suggested red-belted conk mushroom essence for her arthritis, but suggested she stop when it flared into the hot, acute stage.

She began taking the mushroom essence and immediately became angry, along with verbal outbursts and incessant vomiting. I suggested she take one drop in water daily until this passed. By the end of the first month, she had moved up to full dosage and had reduced her Tylenol intake by two-thirds. Another lunar cycle of the same mushroom essence found her relatively pain-free and becoming more flexible and social.

Six months later, she signed up for a bicycle trip in Ireland with her neighbor and nineteen other women, all of similar age. While overseas, she became fascinated with Celtic mythology and stopped her regular weekly church attendance.

TINDER CONK • AMADOU
(Fomes fomentarius)

INDICATIONS: anger, fear, heart, judgment, masculinity

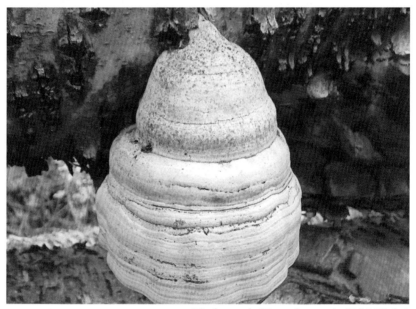

Tinder conk (*Fomes fomentarius* [L.] J. Kickx)

Men weren't really the enemy—they were fellow victims
suffering from an outmoded masculine mystique that made them
unnecessarily inadequate when there were no bears to kill.

—BETTY FRIEDAN

Fomes means to foment, to heat up or burn. The common name amadou is derived from a northern French dialect meaning "amorous" or "inflames life." This derives from the Latin *amare,* and in turn, from French word for "punk." The term *punk* traditionally applied to a prostitute, who sparked her lover into flame. *Spark* and *spunk* (semen) are derivatives.

Ötzi the iceman, whose five-thousand-year-old remains were found in the Alps in 1991, carried a dung water-soaked strip of the context material, from under the outside surface, as a fire starter. The author proudly possesses two unique hats made from the chamois-like material, carefully carved from the inner surface of this polypore.

Tinder conk is commonly found on birch throughout North America, and is one of the most abundant polypores in the boreal forest. The gray color is associated with twilight, or between-the-realms energy.

Our relationship with fire is ancient. The forests renew themselves with fire, and humans rejuvenate with inner fire. The fire element in traditional Chinese medicine is related to the heart, circulation, arteries, and veins.

The word *artery* derives from Ares, the Greek God of War, and relates to Mars, the red planet. The arteries push red oxygenated blood to all parts of the body and represent masculine assertiveness. Venous blood, derived from its relationship to the planet Venus, is passive, blue, and feminine. It is interesting to note, in general, that men have more issues with strokes, hypertension, and aneurisms, while women develop more varicose veins, phlebitis, and related congestive conditions below the waist. This is not a hard and fast rule, just a general observation.

Research has found that children mistreated or exposed to anger as young as six years of age exhibit heart-rate changes. The brain wires itself to this pattern, and this unhealthy pathway becomes stronger. The American Heart Association suggests moderate anger increases arrhythmic heart conditions threefold. Anger throws cardiac rhythm into chaos, with platelets more likely to clot. The heart variability rate is sensitive to these emotional states.

Archetypal patterns find male and female energy can become imbalanced at any age of development. Men must learn to control anger, and women the emotion of fear.

Sam Keen writes:

> *Condition a man [or woman] to value aggression above all other virtues, and you will produce a character type whose most readily expressed emotion will be anger. Condition a woman [or man] to value submission above all other attitudes, and you will produce a character type whose most readily expressed emotion will be sadness.*

Depending upon how you look at it, aggression may be a man's greatest virtue or vice. If our destiny is to conquer and control, it is the prime mover. If our destiny is to live in harmony, it is the legacy of an animal past.... Research has shown that it is not simple aggression but aggression mixed with hostility that predisposes type A personalities to heart attacks.[7]

Research has looked at formation of calcium deposits on the arteries and has found significant correlation between higher levels of hostility and calcification. This may develop into severe atherosclerosis.

Early family dynamics will affect how this pattern plays out, sometimes influencing people all their lives. One example is the high rate of physical assault associated with professional athletes. They have been rewarded, since they were young, for exhibiting and performing violent behavior in their sport.

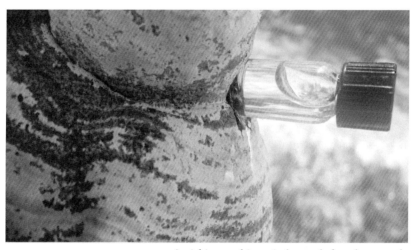

A vial inserted into tinder conk for a lunar cycle

Essence Description

Tinder conk essence helps us reconnect with the spark of life and carry this torch of awareness down into personal relationships.

For the male, anger is often a quick response to a perceived invasion of personal space or confrontation of ideals. For the female, the pattern can become deeply negative as well, showing up in subtle expressions of control and manipulation. In fact, in a Dutch study of 875 patients, type D (depressive) personalities were found to have a fivefold greater risk of dying or experiencing heart attack nine months later.[8] Both patterns, occurring at the same time in a couple relationship, will quickly lead to reactivity, deception, and a death spiral of disconnection.

Tinder conk essence modifies and allows greater expression of masculine and feminine gifts, without judgment of self and others. It helps bring heart-centered attention to what is important, and encourages awareness of how we can move through the world in a more soulful manner.

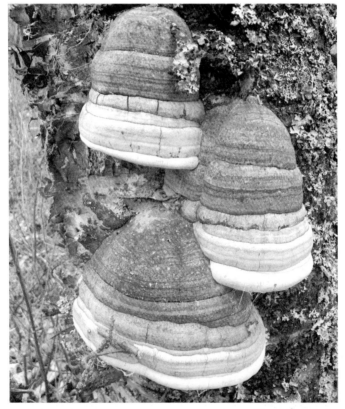

Fomes fomentarius

PREPARATION: This essence is created over a twenty-eight-day cycle from full moon to full moon. A vial of pure rainwater with a small amount of colloidal silver is inserted into the living conk. This is removed after the lunar cycle and combined with an equal part of brandy. It is best prepared under Aries or Leo.

CASE STUDY: Brian was a fifty-five-year-old man, married, with no children. His father died of a heart attack at age fifty-seven. He was experiencing extreme bouts of anger, both verbal and physical. His ECG and cardiograms were normal, and yet the client felt chest pains and palpitations that woke him up several times a night. The first lunar cycle of this mushroom essence made a significant change in heart symptoms and improved his sleep. Recurring dreams involving his father were chaotic and violent. One night, he had a vision of himself as a six-year-old, watching his father physically beat his mother. He awoke in a panicked state. He said to me several times at his next visit, "I am not my father." Shortly thereafter, he entered counseling for anger management.

CHAGA
(Inonotus obliquus)

INDICATIONS: belief, cancer, constriction, self-doubt, pineal gland, pituitary, karma, indoctrination, religion, karma

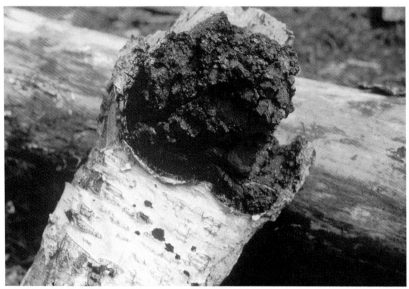

Chaga (*Inonotus obliquus* [Acharius ex Persoon] Pilát)

Even if all the experts agree, they may well be mistaken.

—BERTRAND RUSSELL

It is only in appearance that time is a river. It is rather a vast landscape and it is the eye of the beholder that moves.

—THORNTON WILDER

The word "belief" is a difficult thing for me. I don't believe. I must have a reason for a certain hypothesis. Either I know a thing, and then I know it—I don't need to believe it.

—CARL JUNG

Inos means "fiber," and *noton* means "back." *Oblique* suggests the pores are at an angle to the ground. In fact there are no real pores, as the very rare fruiting body is seldom observed.

Chaga is a sterile conk associated with birch trees. It is an important medicinal mushroom that shows promise in various cancer *miasms*. More study is needed, particularly human clinical trials, to prove efficacy.

The colors are black covering rusty brown. Black represents heaviness, issues of death, decay, and lack of awareness. Rusty brown represents blood, groundedness, instincts, and lower emotions.

Essence Description

Chaga essence is associated with emotional and spiritual constriction, and is useful for individuals whose rigid belief systems have diminished their vitality and energy. Our belief systems are introduced early in life, long before we adopt critical thinking. One belief is tacked upon another, and soon an entire train of indoctrination has left the station.

Jesuit priests say that if you give them access to a child until six years of age, they will practice Catholicism for the rest of their lives. Religious instruction begins early in life so that belief replaces reason, and the brain perceives the ups and downs of life as good or bad, right or wrong, divine or evil. This, in turn, can lead to assumptions or presumptions about our true nature and connection with higher self. Many Christian religions place the higher self or spiritual essence as external to the physical plane. In fact, many indoctrinated people will look skyward when they speak of god or heaven.

For some individuals, belief in a benevolent entity helps fill their lives with more grace and compassion. For others, a vengeful god wracks them with feelings of guilt, sin, and confession. In some cases, these belief systems direct movement toward personal spiritual enlightenment and away from soul development. Religious upbringing is associated with less altruism, according to a recent study published in *Current Biology*.[9]

Spirit is about our heavenly connection, and soul work is digging down to connect with our own unique, individual identity. Meditation and prayer are helpful to connect with spirit but do nothing for soul development. People living excessively in the upper world see light, peace, unity, and love. They aspire to "enlightenment." But everyone, at some time, needs to go underground to complete soul development. Karma can be a self-fulfilling prophecy, with endless loops and twists that bind like a Möbius strip. Karmic debt may be acknowledged and released with chaga mushroom essence.

On a physical level, chaga is one of the richest sources of melanin discovered. Melanin is highly sought by the pineal gland, the third eye. Also known as the sixth chakra, this energy center is associated with inner wisdom. The spirit molecule, or DMT, is produced in the pineal gland and is associated with spiritual ecstasy or enlightenment.

Melatonin helps encourage sleep and reconnection with dreams. The pineal gland is most affected by music therapy, restoring emotional connection with deeper self.

Jack Schwarz writes:

> The pineal is your connection with the transpersonal self and your greatest health/energy state. It transforms light energy in order to make it understandable and usable for you. It is responsible for your being able to transcend into knowingness. But the pineal is never fully functional until all other energy centers and organs are functioning appropriately.... If you allow desire to become part of your whole being, the desire will become strong enough that you will want to express it. Remember, expression is a two-way street. Your radiance, which is determined by your expression, then determines what you attract from the universe, including ideas. Ideas are attracted to you and are initially processed through the pineal gland.[10]

The pineal gland will then energize the gonads and stimulate the energy needed to put an idea into action.

We have all heard the saying, "seeing is believing." One survey found 74 percent of Americans believe angels exist, but only 25 percent believe we evolved from apelike ancestors. When we look to the horizon, we would be led to believe the earth is flat. But when viewed from space, the beauty of our round planetary orb is obvious.

Used in conjunction with cancer therapy, chaga essence may be useful when emotional rigidity is playing a negative role in immune response. That is, the immune system responds to our thoughts, and acts upon them as if they were true. Cancer can open gateways to the soul, and encourage us to ask questions about our true purpose on earth.

The implications are profound—just like self-fulfilling prophecies, the perception that we are well means that we are. The inner dialogue associated with doubt and illness may also manifest if dwelled upon.

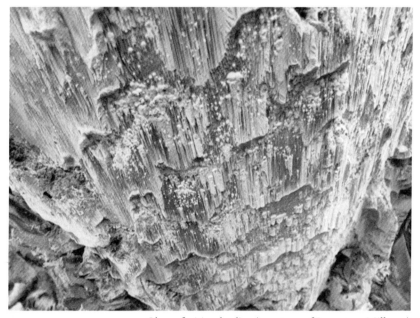

Chaga fruiting bodies (courtesy of Lawrence Millman)

Thomas Moore wrote:

> *Sardello looks at imagery in cancer and concludes that its message is that we live in a world where things have lost their body and therefore their individuality. Our response to this disease could be to abandon the mass culture of plastic reproductions and recover a sensitivity to things of quality and imagination.[11]*

In fact, there are many cases of individuals using imagery to deal with cancer. According to Jack Schwarz, "Whatever you will is synthesized by the pituitary gland, as determined by your health state, beliefs, knowingness, and past experiences, with the final product being sent to the pineal gland. Then the pineal gland integrates the amplitude and frequency of that thought with what is flowing into you from the universe."[12]

Chaga mushroom essence helps create and maintain a vibrational resonance connecting us with universal truths. It helps encourage a reexamination of belief systems and opening up to the possibilities of soul connection.

PREPARATION: Chaga mushroom essence is prepared by drilling a hole in the sterile conk and inserting a sealed test tube of rainwater that contains a small amount of colloidal silver. This is kept in place for an entire lunar cycle, preferably ending with a full moon in Pisces for spirit, or Sagittarius for expanded possibilities. An essence from the fruiting bodies is produced, by placing them on top of rainwater in a crystal bowl, for a single night. These two parts are combined in an equal ratio and stabilized with brandy.

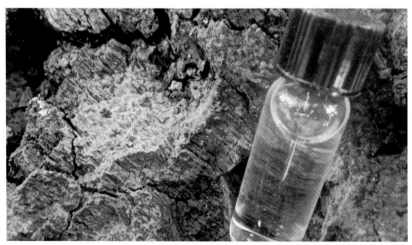

Making mother stock in chaga sterile conk with an inserted water vial.

CASE STUDY 1: Mary was a forty-five-year-old single woman recently diagnosed with breast cancer. She was scheduled for a radical mastectomy, followed by possible radiation and chemotherapy. She appeared in my office extremely timid, shy, introverted, and very passive in her acceptance of the diagnosis. I suggested chaga mushroom essence might be helpful for the emotional aspects of cancer.

She started taking Chaga mushroom essence for one lunar cycle, and almost immediately began to experience, as she put it, an "awakening."

"I have been asleep most of my life," she remarked. By the end of twenty-eight days, her mental attitude had totally shifted. On her next visit, she decided to get a second and then third opinion, resulting in eventually postponing the surgery. She soon began less invasive treatments with a naturopathic colleague.

CASE STUDY 2: Darren was seventy-two years old, widowed, and a retired postal worker. He had recently been diagnosed with high PSA levels, suggestive of prostate cancer. His doctor recommended surgery, but he wanted a second opinion.

We discussed how, in some cases of slow-growing prostate tumors, elderly men often die of something totally unrelated, sometimes twenty or thirty years later. He was fearful of the word *cancer*. A lunar cycle of chaga mushroom essence led him to a renewed determination to examine his options carefully. He declined the surgery, and passed away at age eighty-six from a brain aneurism.

CHICKEN OF THE WOODS
(Laetiporus sulphureus)

INDICATIONS: constriction, distinction, passion, gregariousness, imbalance, introversion, egotism, inspiration, feeling trapped, animation, alchemy

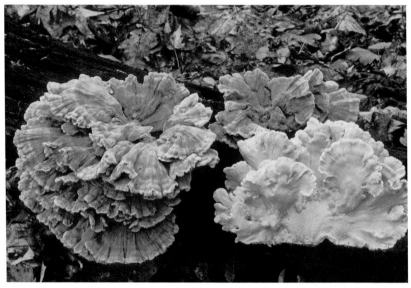

Chicken of the woods (*Laetiporus sulphureus* [Bulliard] Murrill) (courtesy of John Plischke III)

A man who has not passed through the inferno of his passions has never overcome them.
—CARL JUNG

Roast me in Sulphur! Wash me in steep-down gulfs of liquid fire!
—SHAKESPEARE, OTHELLO 1.2

Soul is where the fires of our passions burn.
—BEN SHIELD

Laetiporus is from the Latin, meaning "a wealth of pores." *Sulphureus* alludes to the bright yellow color and rotten-egg smell. In alchemy, the elements mercury, salt, and sulfur interact and form the basis of this philosophical principle. According to Wood:

> *Mercurius is the spirit, that is, the archetypal, pre-material essence from which the outward form is constructed. Sulfur is the mortal soul inhabiting the body. Salt is the body.... Sulfur is the root of "energy-processes" or metabolism in the body. It is the "matchstick" of the body, causing things to burn in order to remove waste materials and promote activity.*[13]

Twentyman contributed to this concept:

> *Sulfur is known to us in nature in six different metamorphic forms, the real elementary, unchanging: sulfur is not a matter of experience; it is the Idea manifesting in these different forms. In the human kingdom this ideal sulfur, which we could also call functional sulfur, manifests through all the metabolic processes. In these it warms and cooks, mixes and pervades it all with a spirit of togetherness or gregariousness. Gregariousness breaks down barriers and distinctions of class and rank. It brings about equality but in the loss of distinctiveness, consciousness is also lost, submerged in the ocean of unconsciousness or sleep consciousness.*[14]

Essence description

Chicken of the woods or sulfur shelf essence is related to the process of heat generation in the body, helping to dissipate or move it when concentrated inappropriately. A cold or flu is an obvious physical condition, but so are flashes of heat associated with perimenopause, andropause, and menopause.

The generation and movement of blood around the body is associated with our connection to the here and now. Alternating hot and cold, or left- and right-sided differences in body temperature, are suggestive of emotional or spiritual imbalance. This may be related to

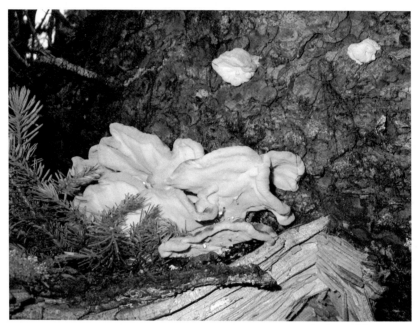

Young chicken of the woods

issues of gender, as the right side of the body is considered masculine, and the left side feminine.

Chicken of the woods mushroom essence relates to inspiration, passion, and the spark of life that inflames infectious enthusiasm. Inspiration involves movement of spirit and creative juices into areas of interest. It helps create gregarious connections, bringing together individuals of like-minded vision.

Chicken of the woods mushroom essence helps individuals who feel trapped in the downside or pressures of life, and envy those who possess charisma and charm. It helps us connect broad horizontal trains of thought into cohesive patterns and systems, and helps us surrender to soul.

When Jung developed a new system of psychoanalysis, his synthesis of objective science and the world of myths and legends changed forever our way of viewing dreams and soul connection. Chicken of the woods helps us tap the unconscious and the hidden wisdom waiting to be uncovered, to move beyond our psychological defenses and into the unknown. The immature ego is selfish, self-important, vain, and conceited; the mature ego is loving and altruistic. A healthy ego is naturally narcissistic and can become lost or stuck when resistant to change.

Chicken of the woods mushroom essence helps us add animation and exuberance into performance, whether through auditory or visual media. It helps us think, feel, and act in a more worldly fashion and leave the minute pieces and details to others.

It is not surprising that it is more useful to the introvert, but it can also be helpful to the boastful and exaggerating extrovert who cannot help but embellish a story for more laughs or greater effect. These individuals are resisting connection to soul and fear loss of ego. They are helped as well by the mushroom essence.

PREPARATION: The mushroom essence is produced overnight from new growth during the waxing of moon or under the influence of Leo. The fresh fruiting body is laid gill-down on rainwater in a crystal bowl.

CASE STUDY: Cynthia was a twenty-two-year-old single woman with a cold, dry, melancholic temperament. She was working in a coffee shop as a barista but wanted to be an artist. She began a lunar cycle of this mushroom essence and reported restlessness and flushes of heat. She began to miss work and felt like sleeping all day. One morning she turned on some music and began to dance around her apartment. She remembered dancing as a child and taking ballet lessons for several years.

One night, she dreamed about a severe reprimand, received from her ballet teacher, when she was eight years old, and in the dream, telling herself she would never dance again. She awoke and began to cry. She realized how much she had denied and repressed her love of dance. She kept her day job and began to take dance classes in the evening.

I did not see her for about six months. The change was dramatic. Now before me stood a radiant, shining being, full of self-confidence and passion.

CINNABAR
(Pycnoporus cinnabarinus)

INDICATIONS: depression, aliens, anger, temper, guilt, dreams, foreboding, shouting, frustration, victimhood, martyrdom, impatience, agitation, time

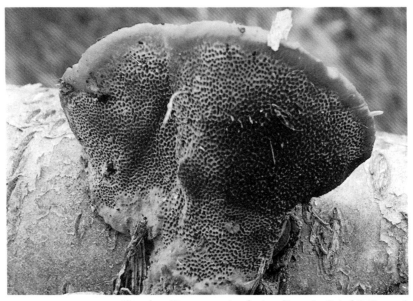

Cinnabar (*Pycnoporus cinnabarinus* [Jacquin: Fries] P. Karsten)

A quick-tempered man does foolish things ... but
a patient man has great understanding.
—PROVERBS 14:17

Impatience is experiencing the moment as empty, useless, meaningless.
—HENRI NOUWEN

Pycnoporus means "many small pores." *Cinnabarinus* is the color, cinnabar red, related to the element mercury, or quicksilver. The powder cinnabar is mercury sulfide (HgS). Cinnabar powders are used in feng shui to expel bad chi and evil spirits, as well as to bring good fortune.

The mineral is produced most often as the result of a volcanic eruption or from a hot spring. Cinnabar drawings more than thirty thousand years old have been found on the walls of caves in Spain and France. Cinnabar comes from the heart (blood) of the earth and opens opportunities for the future.

The name is deceptive, as the polypore is not red but a powerful deep, rich orange. The second chakra responds to the color orange and corresponds to our sexual energy and basic instincts. Ironically, orange clothing is worn in both prisons and monasteries. In Confucianism, the color represents transformation, and indeed, that is its role. In Buddhism, orange represents illumination. It is a color either embraced or loathed.

Individuals helped by cinnabar essence are easily annoyed and frustrated, short-tempered, with a desire to scream and shout. There is impatience with the daily tasks of life and a need for tidiness. Along with irritability is sadness and depression. A spiral of sensitivity to criticism is followed by losing our temper, the desire to be alone, and then depression and loneliness.

We may want to cry, or be sad and angry at the same time. Mistakes and self-doubt are commonly present. A sense of danger is found in dreams, from personal worries to wanting to rescue others. A sense of foreboding and fear may be present upon waking. Dreams of aliens are common. Disorder annoys us. We cannot live in an environment that is not perfectly clean. There may be skin itchiness, or perhaps discomfort from being trapped in our own skin.

Anger is the first emotion learned and the last, for many people, to manage. The Hebrew word for wrath means to "burn with indignation." Many people try to deny, suppress, or pretend anger does not affect them. Turned inward, anger becomes depression or martyrdom. We begin to express "poor me" sentiment and become victims. We excel at creating guilt and unhappiness around us. Martyrdom is a basic character flaw that can become a dominating factor in life.

Impatience may begin in early childhood, when either parent fears a lack of time. The phrase "time is money" may have been spoken and ingrained without thinking. By the age of seven, a child begins to understand that time is in limited supply. In turn, the present moment is not fully enjoyed. An association between rushing and survival is the belief system upon which life is built. They begin to think of the future all the time. Our worst fear is then losing time. "If time is lost, I am lost," is the resulting thought pattern. This essence combines well with varnish conk for issues around time.

Essence description

Cinnabar mushroom essence helps us discern whether our anger is the cause or the symptom. Anger can consume, like the orange flame of fire, with desires of vengeance and thoughts of revenge, even violence. More importantly, anger can create a toxic environment and injure our physical as well as emotional health. Unhealed wounds will fester and remain an irritation. Impatience leads to short temper, intolerance, and a reckless, abrupt, and rude nature. Internally, this can lead to agitation, fretfulness, and eagerness.

One thing many people notice on taking cinnabar mushroom essence is an underlying sense of entitlement. There is a deep-seated belief that we are owed something, and we feel betrayed or indignant when denied what we desire. Or we may play the victim and react, firmly believing our anger is justified. But we have no control over what other people say or do, only our reactions.

Cinnabar mushroom essence teaches that anger is a choice; no one makes us angry. Oftentimes, anger comes to the surface due to feelings of helplessness and frustration. Cinnabar mushroom essence helps teach patience. The Hebrew word for patience means "slow to anger."

Observe, when taking a few drops of the essence in heated moments, and holding it under the tongue for just ten seconds, that a change and shift will take place in the energy pattern surrounding the issue. Patient and uncritical listening changes everything.

Take a look at your wardrobe. How much orange clothing do you own or wear? One of the difficult challenges with anger and irritation is acknowledgment of its existence. Because it is considered impolite, many individuals do not allow themselves to feel its negative influence and suppress it. Injury to the liver and gall bladder can result from long-term expressions of denial and repressed emotion. There is a refusal to allow for soul expansion, but there are constant repeated upheavals on the ego level.

In Christianity the color represents gluttony. Indeed, swallowing our words or feelings can aggravate the liver and gall bladder, leading to bilious attacks of inflammation and pain. Biting the tongue or lip may help reveal this long-standing pattern. Deep-seated and long-standing resentment and the need to control can lead to gallstones and painful episodes involving the gall bladder or pancreas.

Shouting is helpful, but again, in a controlled setting. Find a spot that is special to you and take four to five drops of cinnabar essence under the tongue. Wait patiently for one minute and then shout loudly, again and again, until you have exhausted the energy of the experience. Take four to five drops again and sit peacefully and feel the shift in yourself. This moment gives opportunity for soul connection.

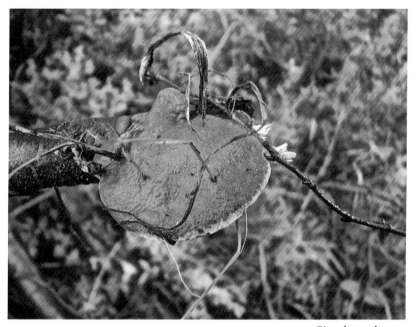

Cinnabar polypore

PREPARATION: The mushroom essence is produced from the fresh fruiting body in rainwater during the influence of the full moon, or when the moon is in Aries.

CASE STUDY: Joseph was a forty-eight-year-old man, married, with four children. He was an insurance broker. He was very obese—five-foot-eight and weighing 280 pounds—with a yellow complexion and deep liver creases between his eyes above the nose.

He came to see me accompanied by his wife. He complained of chronic skin itching. Blood work showed no pathology, but he was constantly scratching his skin, which was bleeding, infected, and irritated. His wife tried to speak several times, but he immediately turned and glared until she became quiet. I asked if he angered easily, and he replied, "Sometimes." I asked if angry outbursts occurred daily, and his wife said, "How about hourly," at which he exploded verbally with an loud angry retort.

I said nothing. I waited in uncomfortable silence until he calmed down. He spoke calmly about how he was constantly frustrated with work and life in general. I asked him if he ever had a bitter taste in his mouth after bouts of anger, to which he replied in the affirmative. I suggested he begin cinnabar mushroom essence in the manner described above. I suggested he take time each day to shout in a controlled environment, as often as needed.

One lunar cycle later, they returned, and he looked very different. He wrote in a dream journal at my request, and mid-month he experienced the identical dream two nights in a row. He was captured by aliens and was traveling through time and space. On the journey, he saw one of the aliens turn into his father. He awoke in a sweat, shivering in fear. His father was a strict, cold, fundamentalist preacher, whom he feared as a child and young adult. He remembered being frustrated as a child, and not being allowed to express himself. I recommended a marriage counselor, whom they contacted the same day.

TURKEY TAIL

(Trametes versicolor)

INDICATIONS: authenticity, relaxation, envy, obsession, criticism

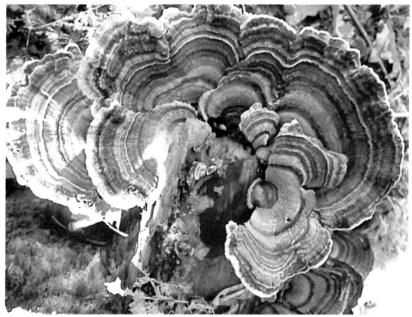

Turkey tail (*Trametes versicolor* [L.] Lloyd)

I kind of view everybody like a rainbow. Everybody on the planet has all the colors of the rainbow inside.
—ALEXIA FAST

This above all: to thine own self be true, And it must follow, as the night the day, Thou canst not then be false to any man.
—SHAKESPEARE, HAMLET 1.3

The authentic self is soul made visible.
—SARAH BAN BREATHNACH

Only the truth of who you are, if realized, will set you free.
—ECKHART TOLLE

Turkey tail is one of our more beautiful mushrooms, revealing every color of the rainbow. In Holland, it is known as fairy bench, and in Germany, butterfly *Trametes*. In mythology, the goddess Iris was Juno's personal messenger, who traveled over the rainbow to reach earth. She probably began as a form of Kali-Maya, a pre-Vedic mistress of the rainbow who shifted reality through her cosmic veils. She was responsible for leading the souls of dead women to the Elysian Fields, the Greek version of heaven. At one time, it was thought that everything was based on rainbows, because strong sunlight would reveal millions of tiny rainbows.

Turkey tail mushroom essence is about feeling comfortable with our true authentic self by supporting and sifting through the cosmic veils of our experience. Catherine Potter, a good friend and fellow faculty member at Northern Star College, shared this saying with me: "What if we never went to a place of having to justify, prove, or defend ourselves again, or put anyone else in that position?"

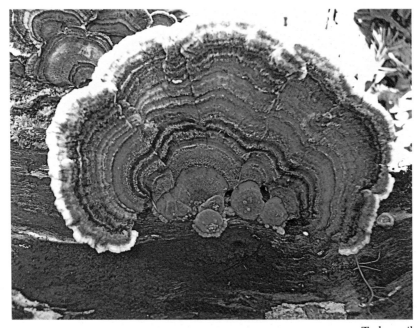

Turkey tail

Essence description

This is the essence of turkey tail. When we view the world from the vantage point of authenticity, experiences become congruent. If we are critical, we will attract criticism. If we operate from a feeling of superiority, this will attract people who enjoy knocking other people off their thrones.

Admiration and obsession with famous people is put into perspective when using turkey tail mushroom essence. Some individuals experience life through the lens of identifying with public or popular media figures. This transference prevents us from attaining personal identification and connection with soul. It is similar to viewing life with our eyes wide open, as opposed to seeing it through a camera lens. In the former case, life is vibrant and robust. The latter creates a two-dimensional aspect that provides superficial avoidance of our own growth.

Living vicariously through a celebrity or our local sports team subjects us to synthetic experiences of emotion, the highs and lows of artificial, once-removed de-attachment. What is happening? This protected observation allows us to envy, despise, or feel familiar with people leading glamorous, exciting lives. Millions of people follow television shows where emotional investment is placed on a singer, or survivor, in hopes of winning a competition. Turning to daily obsessions with favored celebrities as compensation for the feelings of emptiness in our own lives is self-defeating. It prevents nurturance of our own ego and sublimates maturity and soul growth. It is a distraction from soul purpose.

There is another use for turkey tail mushroom essence. Both men and women use false flattery and deception to attract potential mating partners. These encounters are bound to fail due in part to moral and ethical dishonesty. Turkey tail mushroom essence helps us cut through this emotional clutter to find what is honest and true for ourselves. It is an excellent essence to take before meeting someone new for the first time. It wipes clean the contact lenses of intention.

Turkey tail allows us to relax on a physical, mental, and emotional level. It helps us realize the universal connectedness associated with experiencing true self and connection with soul. It allows us to accept criticism for what it is—another opinion.

PREPARATION: The mushroom essence is produced by placing the fruiting bodies pores-down in a crystal bowl of rainwater when the moon is in your solar or lunar sign.

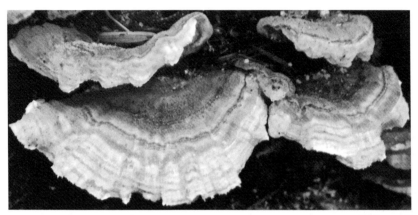

Turkey tail

CASE STUDY: Beth was a forty-five-year-old woman, married, with six children. She complained of lethargy, boredom, and a feeling of emptiness. At my suggestion she began a lunar cycle of turkey tail mushroom essence and kept a dream journal. By mid-cycle she noted her dreams involved social situations with Hollywood movie stars. She was invisible to them, but their activities surrounded her. She realized she had been filling her afternoons with celebrity television talk shows and was living life vicariously through them.

By the end of the lunar cycle, she had separated herself from her addiction to television and began to go for daily walks, which led to her joining a fitness class. For the second lunar cycle, I recommended algae maze. This helped her understand some of her underlying issues, and the difference between aloneness and being lonely. On her last visit she said, "Now when people tell me they are bored, I don't even know what they mean."

MAZE GILL

(Lenzites betulina)

INDICATIONS: crisis of identity, nervous tension, self-identity, solar plexus

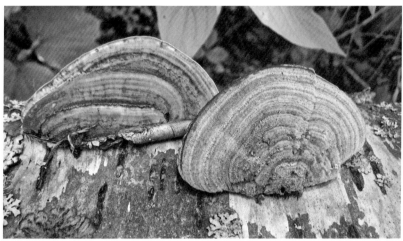

Maze gill or gilled polypore (*Lenzites betulina* [L.] Fries)

The gift you carry for others is not an attempt to save the world,
but to fully belong to it. It's not possible to save the world by
trying to save it. You need to find what is genuinely yours
to offer the world before you can make it a better place.

—BILL PLOTKIN

Gilled polypore, another name for maze gill, is a seeming oxymoron: mushrooms are generally either gilled or pored. It appears that this species evolved millions of years ago as an intermediate form. Many specimens, when they grow older, begin to develop green algae on their upper side.

Essence description

Maze gill mushroom essence is associated with crises of identity. This may be seen in the bigger picture as confusion over self-identity and how we fit in with family, friends, and society as a whole. This essence may be useful for the family "black sheep," the one that never seems to follow the path of the others in the household or even close relatives.

The color orange is most often associated with our second chakra, while green relates more to our solar plexus and heart. Maze gill mushroom essence acts as a bridge between the two chakras whenever a blockage of energy is present. The solar plexus is an energetic center of physiology, as it is related to emotions and psychological discomfort or lack of ease.

Oftentimes, the hero's or heroine's journey of self-discovery begins when they leave home. We encounter a shadowy element of our own unconscious that protects or guards the passage into soul connection. We defeat our demon (the ego) and enter the underworld; if slain or dismembered, we descend into death (the former self). Joseph Campbell called it "a world of unfamiliar yet strangely intimate forces."[15] The shadowy elements know us because they are soul fragments of our previously denied self. Connecting with the dark parts of self helps us connect with their true authentic nature. In turn, this creates the power to manifest.

Located in the center of the chest just under the rib cage, the solar plexus ranges in sensitivity from benign to painful. A direct correlation between sources of nervous tension and irritation can be noted. In some cases, maze gill combines well with wolf lichen for issues involving the solar plexus.

PREPARATION: The mushroom essence is produced under an Aquarian moon with living fruiting bodies, both young and old. The mushrooms are placed gills-up in rainwater in a crystal bowl. At least one fruiting body should cohost algae.

CASE STUDY: Josh was thirty-two years old, single, and a professional engineer. He was the oldest of four children in his family, always feeling like the black sheep and never knowing why. He felt estranged from his parents and siblings.

At my recommendation, he began a lunar cycle of maze gill mushroom essence and started a dream journal. He initially found his sleep disrupted, so he reduced the dosage. In about the third week he awoke in the middle of night, startled, with the word *adopted* running through his mind. He felt pain in his solar plexus, as if he were having a heart attack. He began to perspire profusely and could not rise without dizziness.

Several days later he made an impromptu visit to his parents and confronted them about this remote possibility. They confirmed his intuition, which was followed by an emotional catharsis, chaos, and consternation. This was the start of his healing—and theirs.

BIRCH POLYPORE
(Piptoporus betulinus)

INDICATIONS: anxiety, appreciation, depression, envy, melancholy, grace, inertia, pioneering

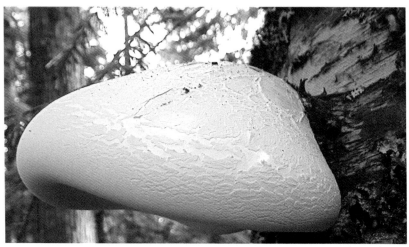

Birch polypore (*Piptoporus betulinus* [Bulliard] P. Karsten)

The trouble with normal is, it always gets worse.
—BRUCE COCKBURN

Every normal person, in fact, is only normal on average.
His ego approximates to that of the psychotic in some
part or other and to a greater or lesser extent.
—SIGMUND FREUD

Depression is the inability to construct a future.
—ROLLO MAY

Birch polypore is an annual fruiting body found exclusively growing with birch. It has a number of interesting medicinal uses and was found with 5,300-year-old Ötzi the iceman. Some authors suggest it is edible, so I found some small ones, cut them thinly, and fried them in butter and garlic. They tasted exactly like a garlic and butter eraser. Some individuals cut small strips and age them for six months or more, then add them to their smoking mixtures. Much better.

Essence description

Birch polypore essence is suited to the explorer, pioneer, trailblazer, and groundbreaker in whichever field we choose. This solitary path is often fraught with challenges, and many individuals become scarred through the difficulties of the journey. However, by overcoming these external and internal challenges, the pioneer undergoes inner transformation.

Birch polypore essence helps these brave souls open opportunity for those who follow. One of the dangers of being ahead of today's popular curve or wave is the feeling of under-appreciation by the social elite and lack of rewards from financial circles. This can lead to melancholy and depression on the personality level. The expectation of receiving acknowledgment from strangers is a futile pursuit.

Birch polypore essence brings lightness and grace to those who have long labored at projects that fulfill their soul purpose. That is the reward. Birch polypore mushroom essence helps ground us on the path chosen, and the soul-centered rewards far surpass any temporary materialism.

It is generally accepted that any new idea has to pass through one or two generations before acceptance by the status quo. Remember this motto: if you do something important, there will always be critics. If you don't like critics, don't do anything important.

Birch polypore essence helps us to feel less restless and anxious and more content on a day-to-day basis. Relaxation and greater understanding of issues around envy or jealousy will occur. Judgment on people who have chosen a more traditional or conventional life path will begin to vanish. Birch polypore essence is a teacher of limitations, from highs and lows.

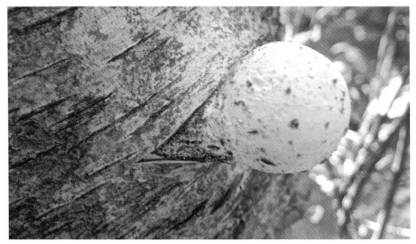

Young birch polypore

Birch polypore essence helps us accept that normal is highly over-rated and can, for some individuals, lead to anxiety, melancholy, depression, and inertia. In fact, many psychologists attempt to fit clients into a "normal" world through behavioral adjustment and superficial mind alterations. Jungian psychologists and like-minded mental health practitioners do not work with behavioral modification. Some psychologists believe that depression is simply anger turned inward. Moore writes:

> *Depression may be as important a channel for valuable "negative" feelings as expressions of affection are for the emotions of love. Feelings of love naturally give birth to gestures of attachment. In the same way, the void and grayness of depression evoke an awareness and articulation of thoughts otherwise hidden behind the screen of lighter moods.*[16]

Melancholy and depression both contain a layer of sadness. The former suggests a longing to see things in a different light. Depression can lead to inaction and withdrawal. Fear can move us from melancholy to depression when we fail to find meaning in our sadness. Moore continues:

> *Today, we seem to prefer the word depression over sadness and melancholy.... But there was a time, five or six hundred years ago,*

when melancholy was identified with the Roman god Saturn. To be depressed was to be "in Saturn," and a person chronically disposed to melancholy was known as a "child of Saturn."[17]

To be saturnine suggests we are cold and steady in mood, or slow to act or change. In medical terms it refers to absorption of lead in the system. Saturn return is an astrological transit that occurs when the planet returns to the same place in the sky that it occupied when we were born. It occurs every twenty-eight or twenty-nine years, the first return signaling the movement from youth to adulthood. The second, at age fifty-six to fifty-nine, is associated with midlife crisis. For these issues, combine with badia and honey mushroom essences.

Moore expands the issue of depression and melancholia:

One advantage of using the traditional image of Saturn, in place of the clinical term depression, is that then we might see melancholy more as a valid way of being rather than as a problem that needs to be eradicated.… Saturn was also traditionally identified with the metal lead, giving the soul weight and density, allowing the light, airy elements to coalesce. In this sense, depression is a process that fosters a valuable coagulation of thoughts and emotions.[18]

Birch polypore essence helps us to accept the stages of emotion that surround soul connection. Our souls are neither inside us nor outside. They are our true selves.

PREPARATION: The mushroom essence is produced by inserting a vial of rainwater with a small amount of colloidal silver into a young fruiting body in late spring and leaving it for a full lunar cycle. The mature fruiting body is an annual and realizes full potential in a single summer. Starting and ending under the influence of Capricorn is optimal.

CASE STUDY: Robin was a thirty-nine-year-old single holistic practitioner. He enjoyed his work with clients but suffered periods of depression and melancholy. He admitted to being a dreamer and futurist and was frustrated with the lack of progress toward integrative medicine. At my suggestion, he began taking birch polypore essence, and quickly

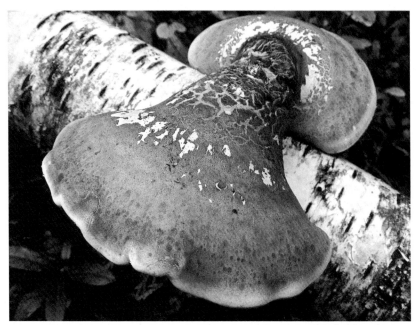

Twin birch polypores

found himself becoming weepy and teary. After five days, this changed to a period of confusion, and he began questioning his own belief systems. However, he continued taking the mushroom essence for the remainder of the lunar cycle.

The same essence was suggested for a second cycle, but combined with cinnabar mushroom essence. Quickly his mood shifted to anger and recognition of an older belief system in which he felt he was owed something. He realized that his work with others was his attempt to please and heal others, so that in turn he would be recognized, acknowledged, and loved. His melancholy gradually shifted and was replaced with gratitude and inspiration. He met his future wife and soul mate less than three months later.

ROSY CONK

(Fomitopsis cajanderi)

INDICATIONS: chastity, sexuality, congestion, constriction, tantra, pain, inflammation, enlightenment, lust

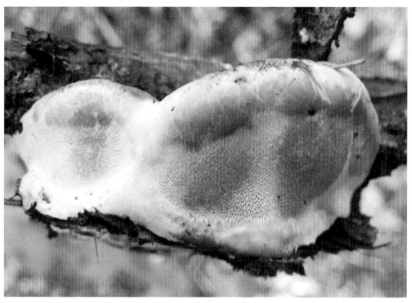

Rosy conk (*Fomitopsis cajanderi* [P. Karsten] Kotlaba & Pouzar)

Whether we fall by ambition, blood, or lust, like
diamonds we are cut with our own dust.

—JOHN WEBSTER

Chastity—the most unnatural of all the sexual perversions.

—ALDOUS HUXLEY

We may eventually come to realize that chastity
is no more a virtue than malnutrition.

—ALEX COMFORT

Rosy conk is a perennial polypore, with vivid pink coloring on the pore side.

Essence description

Rosy conk mushroom essence relates to issues surrounding chastity and lust. Note the beautiful pink-violet color of the fruiting body. Pink is associated with vulnerability and love, two aspects that create confusion around these issues. Violet is associated with our third eye, or sixth chakra.

A number of religions associate abstinence from sex with the pursuit of higher consciousness. This is associated with the belief that the afterlife, or heaven, is an awaited nirvana. Intimacy outside of marriage is considered a sin by some religions. In fact, sexual union *is* heaven on earth and creates a deep-seated connection with our higher selves. Western society tends to isolate sexuality from the totality of nature.

Bill Plotkin writes, "In addition to arousal, coitus, and orgasm, sexual desire can guide us to something more: soul.... Our sexuality, when fully honored, stirs our most creative juices and urges us to cross into the mysteries of nature and psyche."[19]

A good example of sexual distortion is the abstinence required of Roman Catholic priests. The repression of this basic instinct can be linked to men of cloth sexually abusing children, to which the church in turn turned a blind eye. Kathleen Taylor, a neurologist at Oxford University, suggests that we will soon be treating religious fundamentalism and other forms of ideological beliefs potentially harmful to society as a form of mental illness.[20]

Rosy conk mushroom essence is useful for individuals who have turned away from sexual union as part of their desire for spiritual enlightenment. The essence will enhance the enjoyment associated with tantric sex, and allow us the freedom to relax around the need to avoid orgasm. In fact, this restriction of release may be detrimental to the spiral upward movement of kundalini energy throughout the body over the long term.

The mushroom essence allows us to explore our sexuality without inhibition and to simply marvel in the pleasure associated with letting go. This helps us connect and alters our consciousness by pulling us down toward soul.

Rosy conk essence helps us connect with constriction on various chakra levels and dissipate congestion and associated inflammation and pain in the urogenital tract. This includes salpingitis, orchitis, chronic vaginitis, and painful intercourse.

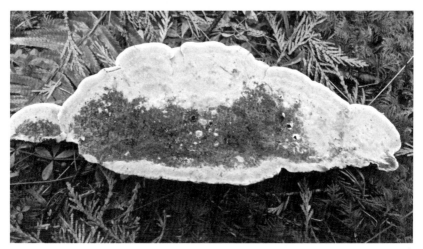

Rosy conk

PREPARATION: Rosy Conk essence is prepared by placing the fruiting body pores-down on top of rainwater in a crystal bowl, ideally when the moon is in Virgo.

CASE STUDY: Vanessa was a twenty-four-year-old single woman working as a dental hygienist. She grew up in a very religious household, attending mass on a weekly basis with her family. She suffered from vaginismus, a painful condition experienced during intercourse. The pain prevented the use of tampons, which were too aggravating to insert. She had dated a few times, but sex was too painful, resulting in short-term relationships with men. Oral sex and masturbation did not help her achieve orgasm.

She took rosy conk mushroom essence and kept a dream journal for one lunar cycle. She found she began to have very erotic dreams, and awoke one morning, shocked to find herself in the midst of self-pleasure. This was deeply disturbing for her, and she stopped taking the mushroom essence.

On her next visit, I recommended she combine it with split gill mushroom essence for a full lunar cycle. She was reluctant, but said she was willing to give it a try. About ten days later, she awoke in the middle of the night to find herself masturbating and shaking violently with orgasmic contractions. This crisis changed the manner of her vaginal contractions to the point she was able to have intercourse, without pain, about eight months later.

IQMIK

(Phellinus igniarius)

INDICATIONS: self-criticism, conditional love, disintegration, trust, fear of success

Iqmik is found growing on birch trees. In Alaska and Yukon, indigenous peoples burn the polypore to ash and add it to tobacco and smoking mixtures. It appears to increase delivery of nicotine to the brain, increasing the activity of brain neurons.

Recent medicinal mushroom studies suggest benefit against influenza viruses A and B and the H1N1, H3N2, and H9N2 strains, as well as amelioration of symptoms associated with multiple sclerosis.

It should not be mistaken for the similar looking *Phellinus tremulae* growing on poplar trees; see the *P. tremulae* image below.

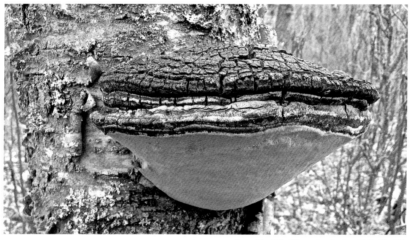

Iqmik (*Phellinus igniarius* [L.] Quél)

Much protective self-criticism stems from growing up around people who wouldn't or couldn't love you, and it's likely they still can't or won't.

—MARTHA BECK

Essence description

Iqmik fungal essence is associated with patterns of self-deprecation and fear of success. How did this pattern begin, and what steps led to this dysfunction and lack of trust and belief in the self? Work by José Stevens in *Transforming Your Dragons* gives great insight into this common yet destructive pattern:

STEP ONE. Children learn that love in their home is conditional.

STEP TWO. Children fear being inadequate, don't know how to change, and identify with being inadequate.

STEP THREE. They apologize for everything and begin to feel unworthy. This leads to always apologizing or saying "sorry" before doing or saying anything.

STEP FOUR. They learn to make themselves small and invisible. They hide well, so that people will not have expectations of them.

STEP FIVE. They begin to predict ahead of time that they will not succeed, as their one sure way to be right about something. "This begins a downward, negative spiral because the children actually search for ways to hide, to be mediocre, and to veer away from leadership."[21]

STEP SIX. Children learn to criticize and put themselves down.

STEP SEVEN. Children learn to avoid success at all costs. This would raise other people's expectations, and when they fail, they would have to go through the discomfort of feeling inadequate again. They decide it is best not to start, leading to the fear-of-success syndrome.

These patterns can lead to a blackness of emotion and personality. Self-destructive tendencies can result, leading to aloneness and loneliness. Iqmik often combines well with algae maze mushroom essences. Dreams of the dead, death, and dying may occur or already be present. In fact, the death of ego at each step of the above cycle can lead to exaggerated pain and discomfort.

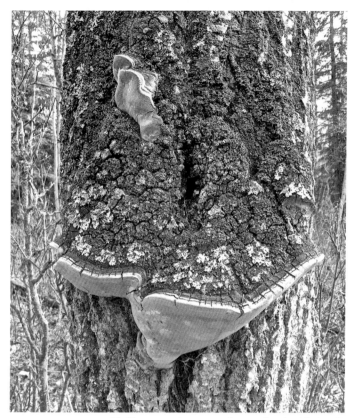

Phellinus tremulae, not to be confused with iqmik

Iqmik mushroom essence should be taken with care, as unveiling deep-seated belief systems can be fracturing and disintegrating. But it is one more step on the path to soul connection. Iqmik mushroom essence works well with vision fasts and quests, in which the ego deconstructs enough that going back to the old way of life is no longer possible.

PREPARATION: This fungal essence is produced by putting a thin layer of the burned ash of the fruiting body on top of rainwater in a crystal bowl. The ash is produced by burning the polypore under anaerobic conditions. A closed can on a bed of coals works well. The full moon is best, but the new moon in Taurus, Virgo, or Capricorn can also work well.

CASE STUDY: Jeff was thirty-three years old, a new and used car sales-man, married, with one child. He was very insecure, suicidal, and self-critical. He indulged in self-reprimands and blamed others for his lack of success in business and marital life. Childhood was filled with conditional love, feeling inadequate, and being unable to please his mother or father.

Jeff began iqmik mushroom essence and noted increased feelings of irritation in his work environment and around his spouse. Dreams of death and dying occurred nightly, and angry outbursts became a common occurrence. He stopped the essence for a time and felt more relaxed but emotionally flat. He started it once more after about six weeks and realized one evening that he was settling for less in his life. He discussed it with his wife and then quit his job, not knowing what was next. Two months later, they were introduced to a multi-level marketing product they could run as a home business from their phone and computer. One year later, they had generated income over $300,000 and were excited and brimming with confidence. Everything changed for the whole family.

BADIA

(Polyporus badius)

INDICATIONS: boredom, empty nest syndrome, self-pity, stagnation

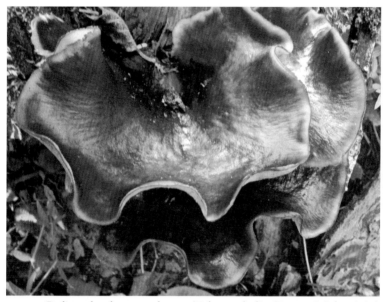

Badia or bay brown polypore (*Polyporus badius* [Persoon] Schweinitz)

There are no second acts in American lives.
—F. Scott Fitzgerald

*Midlife is the time to let go of an over-dominant ego and to
contemplate the deeper significance of human existence.*
—Carl Jung

Badia relates to emotional flexibility. R. C. Peck suggested there are
four psychological advances critical to successful adjustment in middle adulthood:[22]

1. Socializing versus sexualizing in human relationships: redefine the men and women in our lives so that we value them as individuals, friends, and companions, rather than primarily sex objects.

2. Valuing wisdom versus valuing physical powers: wisdom is the capacity to make wise choices in life to compensate for decreases in stamina, physical strength, and youthful attractiveness.

3. Emotional flexibility versus emotional impoverishment: emotional flexibility is the capacity to shift emotional investments from one activity to another and from one person to another.

4. Mental flexibility versus mental rigidity: most people have completed their formal education and have been sufficiently trained for their jobs or careers. They also become set in their ways and closed to new ideas.

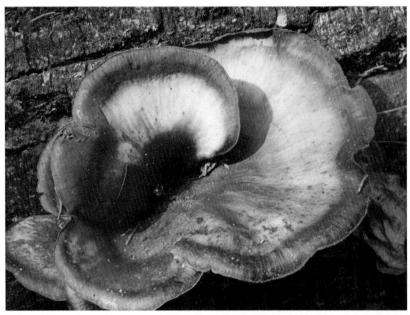

Badia

Essence description

Badia mushroom essence relates specifically to the third issue of emotional flexibility. This may affect men or women of any age, but more often than not, it manifests in early to late middle age. Very often, the so-called midlife crisis is associated with life events such as job loss, financial problems, or illness rather than the natural process of aging. Legal separation and divorce rates peak for males in the forty to forty-four age range. One longitudinal study of more than two thousand adults found few midlife crises and improved personal relationships but less control over sex lives and children.

The midlife crisis is really a midlife consciousness. It is the refusal to hear the call of the soul and returns those who refuse to listen to egocentric refrains of unrewarding work, culture, and relationships. The learned qualities of thankfulness, forgiveness, and empathy are more fully developed. Stagnation, or a sense of boredom, is a self-centered consequence of emotional impoverishment. This may be related to a feeling of inadequate achievement of expected goals. Psychosomatic illness, loss of purpose, and monotony can become problematic.

Badia mushroom essence helps us deal with frustration and self-pity. It helps give us a sense of self-renewal and the continued opportunity for soul-based, personal development.

Badia mushroom essence helps ease the emotional pain of women suffering from empty-nest syndrome. Children have moved out of the family home and are learning their own soul-based lessons as adolescents and young adults. Over-concern and worry for their well-being and happiness can become obsessive.

Badia mushroom essence helps the crone recognize the joy of newly acquired freedom associated with diminished responsibilities. This lends itself to an opportunity to spread our wings and redefine self. Psyche was the goddess and personification of the soul, appearing in the form of a butterfly. Jungian psychology is about connecting us with soul, or our true self. That is the purpose of badia.

PREPARATION: Badia mushroom essence is produced by pouring pristine rainwater into the naturally inverted caps for a full moon night in Gemini or Virgo, and the next day preserving the water one-to-one with brandy.

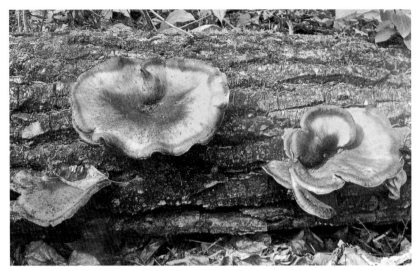

Badia: note the perfect chalices for essence preparation.

CASE STUDY: Holly was a fifty-seven-year-old retail clerk, married for thirty-two years but recently separated. She and her husband had been clients of mine for nine years. She was entering her second full Saturn return.

She was feeling guilty and suffering remorse over a spontaneous affair with her boss. When she confessed this betrayal to her husband, he became angry, upset, and moved out. She came to me feeling despondent, that her life was over. She regretted the affair and recognized that it was due to a lack of excitement in herself, and to the worry that life was passing her by. She began a course of badia mushroom essence, and within ten days had a profound catharsis in which she realized how much she loved and missed her husband. She phoned him, and he agreed to meet at a neighborhood café. He came to the restaurant a few minutes late, carrying a bouquet of twenty-four red roses. Over the next six months, they "dated," she left her job, and he was invited back into their home.

AGARIKON

(Laricifomes officinalis) (Fomitopsis officinalis)

INDICATIONS: dreams, floods, faith, spirituality, water, rebirth

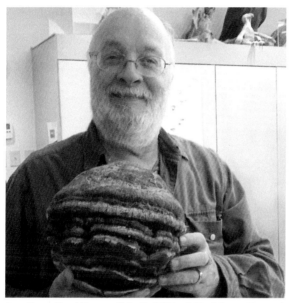

Agarikon (*Laricifomes officinalis* [Villars] Kotlaba & Pouzar)

Water is the commonest symbol for the unconscious. The lake in the valley is the unconscious, which lies, as it were, underneath consciousness, so that it is often referred to as the "subconscious," usually with the pejorative connotation of an inferior consciousness. Water is the "valley spirit," the water dragon of Tao, whose nature resembles water—a yang in the yin, therefore, water means spirit that has become unconscious.

—CARL JUNG

Water is the driving force of all nature.

—LEONARDO DA VINCI

Nothing is softer or more flexible than water, yet nothing can resist it.

—LAO TZU

Agarikon has been used as medicine for several millennia. It is ancient and possesses wisdom associated with this longevity. Dioscorides called this polypore the female agaric, while *Fomes fomentarius,* the tinder conk, was known as the male agaric.

Water is a universal symbol of mystery and the unconscious. Jung understood that water represented emotion, that instead of being composed of air, it becomes a flowing liquid. The spirit becomes water when the dreamer is not able to connect with inner life or soul development. Water is heavy and confined to earth; spirit is light and can go anywhere.

The Christian ritual of baptism involves immersion into water to become "born again." This is a symbol of the descent of consciousness into the unconscious and the resulting new and fuller life. In the Roman Catholic tradition, bread wafers and wine are offered as symbols of the body and blood of Jesus Christ. First Nations groups of the Pacific Northwest call this polypore "the bread of ghosts." The large fruiting bodies were carved into totem animals and strategically positioned to protect a shaman's home and later his grave.

Flood mythology is the first stage of the process of individuation. Noah, from the Judeo-Christian tradition, and Markandeya, from the Hindu tradition, are symbols of this individuation. The flood water—the unconscious—destroys the persona, the self-image we create for ourselves in early adulthood. This partial self must be dissolved to make way for appearance of the whole, soul-connected self.

In some cultures, there is mythology of a diver going to the bottom of the ocean and bringing up treasure. Again, water is the symbol of the unconscious, and the treasure is the new self. Previously unused psychic resources are given appropriate expression in our conscious life.

Water is often the first stage in an insect's life cycle. A dragonfly larva, for example, is like the unconscious sleeping soul, living underwater. At some point it rises to the surface and the soul wakes up. It then transforms and grows wings. The human soul is similar, and once awareness has been attained, it cannot imagine going back to the larval, or unconscious, stage of life. Carl Jung notes, "It is the world of water, where all life floats in suspension; where the realm of the sympathetic system, the soul of everything living, begins."[23]

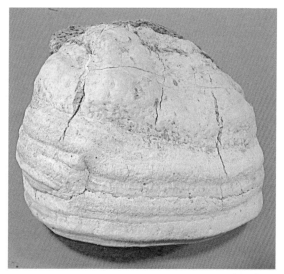

Agarikon

Essence description

Agarikon mushroom essence helps us to deeply reexamine our connection with the dream state. Every ninety minutes during sleep, we have a dream. We dip our toes into the soul stream of consciousness. Keeping a journal will help collect fragments of dreams, and then we can begin to explore their soulful levels of wisdom.

Fear of water, the unconscious, suggests an unwillingness to explore self. It has been suggested by many that the life unexamined is not worth living. Be that as it may, agarikon mushroom essence brings a sense of urgency and vitality to the idea of rebirth. Plotkin writes, "Dreams arise from the waters of our deepest human nature.... The earth, every day, invites us to dive into her dream stream."[24] Agarikon helps us to initially dip our toes, and in time, take a plunge into soul integration.

Agarikon mushroom essence is useful to individuals undergoing shamanic soul retrieval.

PREPARATION: Prepare the same way as chaga: Drill a hole into a live conk. Place a container with fresh rainwater and a small amount of colloidal silver into the opening, and leave it for one lunar cycle. It is best prepared under the influence of a water sign—Pisces, Cancer, or Scorpio.

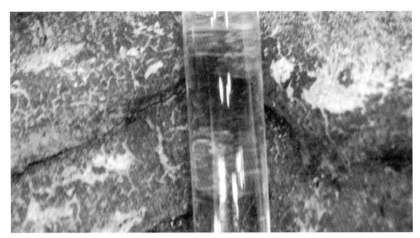

Agarikon with inserted water vial

CASE STUDY: Brittany was twenty-six years old and a PhD student in medical pathology. She had a profound fear of water and believed she had a water allergy. She would not swim or bathe in tubs and was frightened of thunderstorms. She was experiencing terrifying dreams of drowning.

She was highly skeptical of mushroom essences but had been with a behavioral psychotherapist for four years, with little success. The first day she took agarikon essence, she began to cry for the first time in many years. She had lost her mother when she was six years old and had not fully grieved. I suggested she stop taking the mushroom essence for a while. She came for her next appointment three months later and was more relaxed. She was taking baths and was even considering swimming lessons. Four years later, she began taking scuba lessons, and later went to the Caribbean to swim in the ocean with her new fiancé.

BLUE ALBATRELLUS

(Albatrellus flettii)

INDICATIONS: exuberance, feeling overwhelmed, romantic feelings, criticism, femininity, self-fulfilling prophecy, optimism, pessimism, introversion, martyrdom, gloominess

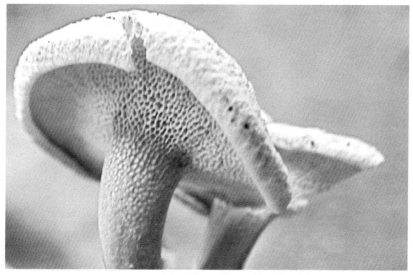

Blue Albatrellus (*Albatrellus flettii* Morse ex Pouzar)

There is no blue without yellow and without orange.
—*VINCENT VAN GOGH*

A pessimist sees the difficulty in every opportunity; an optimist sees the opportunity in every difficulty.
—*WINSTON CHURCHILL*

A pessimist asks you if there is milk in the pitcher; an optimist asks you to pass the cream.
—*OLD SAYING*

The prevailing mood in positive psychology is that optimism is better for health, and an entire industry revolves around positive-thinking books, seminars, and conferences. Pessimism and optimism come in different flavors. Dispositional attitude, for example, is about a chronic tendency to see the glass half full versus half empty. Explanatory attitude is about explaining why bad things happen, with pessimists blaming themselves and optimists blaming external factors. Defensive pessimists will lower expectations and think through all the possible negatives that could happen to help avoid them. Sarah Dessen notes, "If you expect the worst, you'll never be disappointed."[25] True, and some of our great modern comedians rely on humor with a sharp, pessimistic edge.

Medical doctors use the term *hanging crepe*. It means that they give the patient the worst-case scenario and are then seen as heroes when the patient is rescued. They are taught that it is unethical to give hope, despite the fact that a placebo is effective in 30 to 50 percent of cases.

Optimists, when confronted with anxiety-creating events, tend to distract themselves. A recent study in the journal *Psychology and Aging* found that older people with pessimistic views of the future are more likely to live longer and healthier lives.[26] Suzanne Segerstrom, author of *Breaking Murphy's Law,* found optimists "absolutely have an edge in general well-being."[27] Dilip Jeste, who authored a study on optimism in older adults, noted that "being less bothered by stresses can help in coping."[28] He adds that pessimism can be a self-fulfilling prophecy. If we expect the worst, it may happen.

On the other hand, optimism may be a disadvantage in stressful conditions. In a study of 250 couples, overly optimistic people coped worse with stress. The study's coauthor, Erin O'Mara, noted, "Pessimism, to the extent that it allows you to accurately assess what's happening in your life, is important."[29] Thomas Friedman writes, "Pessimists are usually right, and optimists are usually wrong, but all the great changes have been accomplished by optimists."[30]

Essence description

Blue Albatrellus mushroom essence is related to heart-centered feminine qualities, and pessimism, in both sexes. These individuals have a very good nature, are truly genuine, and may be taken advantage of by others. They may be termed "hopeless romantics." At times, they can be overwhelmed by emotions and become gloomy and introverted. Part of their personality predicts and expects the worst, leading to self-fulfilling prophecies. They react poorly to any criticism, but are very kind-hearted, understanding, and forgiving. They generally keep their troubles to themselves, unless prompted to share by people they love.

Blue Albatrellus types may unwittingly become martyrs, sacrificing themselves for others without a full understanding of the implications. The mushroom essence combines well with Cordyceps.

The color blue is calm and clear, suggesting avoidance of issues that may "stir the pot." Blue Albatrellus relates to the benefits of pessimism. As discussed above, some experts believe pessimism is beneficial to physical and mental well-being and may even improve longevity.

Blue Albatrellus mushroom essence helps shift and reshift our internal dialogue in favor of appropriate response to any external stimuli. It helps us to see, feel, and hear from a more soulful reflection and to understand. It helps us to process external stimuli with less judgment and reactivity, allowing for a more detached, heart-centered response.

PREPARATION: Blue Albatrellus essence is produced on a moonlit night under the influence of Capricorn. The fruiting body is layered on top of rainwater in a crystal bowl.

CASE STUDY: Caitlin was a sixteen-year-old high school student. She was brought into my clinic by her mother; concerned about her daughter's moods, withdrawal, and pessimistic attitude. I suggested it is okay to be skeptical, and seeing the glass half empty is better than completely empty. Both mother and daughter were uncertain, but she agreed to try blue Albatrellus mushroom essence for one lunar cycle.

I didn't see her again for eighteen months, but then I received a call from her mother, thanking me. She told me that while taking the mushroom essence, her daughter awoke one night with the frightening memory of her father entering her bed when she was six years old. The story unfolded, and she continued to make progress with a psychotherapist.

ALGAE MAZE POLYPORE
(Cerrena unicolor)

INDICATIONS: aloneness, loneliness, neuroses, psychoses, isolation, womb, arrogance, obsessive-compulsive disorder (OCD), attention deficit hyperactivity disorder (ADHD)

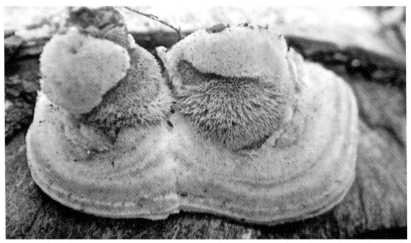

Algae maze polypore (*Cerrena unicolor* [Bulliard] Murrill)

What a lovely surprise to finally discover
how unlonely being alone can be.
—ELLEN BURSTYN

All men's misfortunes spring from their hatred of being alone.
—JEAN DE LA BRUYÈRE

The time you feel lonely is the time you most need to be by yourself.
—DOUGLAS COUPLAND

The common name is due to the growth of algae on top of mature polypores. Mossy maze is another commonly used name, but there is no moss involved. Maze relates to the distinct convoluted structures on the underside of the mushroom.

Essence description

Algae maze essence relates to conditions of aloneness and loneliness. These are two different mental and emotional patterns, but they are linked. The latter is a feeling of isolation, that our expectations are not being met. It is a seeking, a craving for something missing inside us. Aloneness is the freedom to be content in our own company. It is an awareness that we are complete, whole, and connected to life. Loneliness is a state of suffering, because something or someone is missing. Loneliness is a state of mind, and alone is a state of being. Alone is the opportunity to know ourselves, and loneliness is finding company with someone else. Aloneness is contracted and yang; loneliness is more expansive and yin.

Jung wrote, "Loneliness does not come from having no people about one, but from being unable to communicate the things that seem important to oneself, or from holding certain views which others find inadmissible.... If a man knows more than others, he becomes lonely."[31] And arrogant—the attitude of superiority and rude dismissal of those individuals with physical or mental difficulties creates isolation. They then learn to justify their self-imposed isolation through strictly intellectual internal dialogue.

We are social beings, and need to be seen for who we are, if only by one other person. It is not uncommon for individuals to attract like-minded partners, but this is no soul-connected relationship, rather a means of reinforcing a dysfunctional, empty journey of distraction. Loneliness may relate to remembering a time of connection, such as being in our mother's womb. Thousands of people have remembered their intrauterine existence and the traumatic experience of birthing.

Loneliness can motivate us to move out of one state of mind into another. It can turn destructive when an escape from reality leads to distractive activity. Plotkin writes, "The uninitiated ego, with knowledge of the soul's world, has little choice but to project all of its longing onto an outer human beloved. Its loneliness continuously fuels the desire for love affairs."[32] This is common. We are fearful about feeling our own body sensations, leading to denial and stress. Loneliness turned inward can lead to depression and despair that life will not change. It is a form of arrogance, for how can we know the future?

Aloneness helps us to enjoy life in a complete manner, not dependent on money, cars, food, or sex. It can turn negative, in the case of loners, and may become pathological, neurotic, obsessive-compulsive, or even psychotic. Tobacco addiction is six times higher in individuals with psychoses. But which creates which? Combine with earth star for issues surrounding nicotine addiction.

Obsessive-compulsive behavior, or any addictive behavior, is an attempt to shut out unpleasant mental or emotional feelings. It is a ritual of defending a vulnerable personality from pain, but may lead to arrogance or self-satisfaction. Neither is bad nor good. In some situations, it combines well with giant puffball.

Algae maze mushroom essence helps us to meditate more easily and find the proper balance of calmness from within. The mushroom essence assists with the process of understanding our needs and desires in a natural and soul-centered manner.

For tendencies to arrogance, it combines well with oyster mushroom essence.

PREPARATION: Algae maze essence is produced by pouring rainwater on the maze gills of overturned polypores. They are left overnight on or approaching a full moon in either of the water signs Cancer or Aquarius. In the morning, combine one-to-one with brandy.

CASE STUDY: Matt was a thirty-two-year-old single chemical engineer. He was diagnosed with attention deficit disorder (ADD) in fourth grade and had been taking the prescription drug Ritalin for twenty-four years. He initially exhibited a lot of boastful bravado, but before our session was over, he admitted to feeling lonely. We explored this issue and talked about aloneness and loneliness. He said he had no close friends and suffered great difficulty around asking women for dates. In fact, he had stopped dating, as it had become too terrifying to risk rejection.

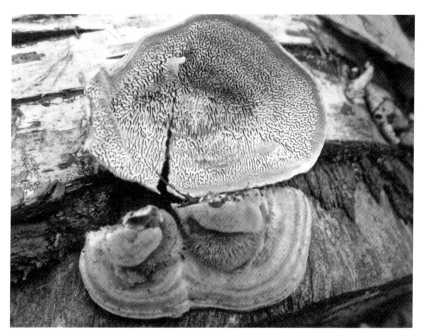

Algae maze

He agreed to try algae maze mushroom essence and took it, as suggested, for a whole lunar cycle. He reported at the next session that he felt more relaxed and was enjoying his alone time much more. I saw him three months later. He began taking yoga classes and was meditating daily. He had dated two different women and admitted to feeling less anxiety around the opposite sex.

DIAMOND WILLOW FUNGUS

(Haploporus odorus)

INDICATIONS: courage, foolishness, contrariness, transparency, protection, shadow work, soul, vision quests, crying, fasting rituals

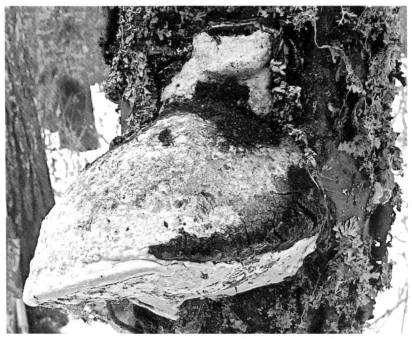

Diamond willow fungus (*Haploporus odorus* [Sommerfelt] Bondartsev & Singer) (courtesy of Kelly Harlton)

The whole man is challenged and enters the fray with his total reality. Only then can he become whole and only then can God be born.

—CARL JUNG

It is the longing that does all the work.

—RUMI

Cree shamans and healers of northern Canada smudge this prized fungus for blessings as part of cleansing and empowerment ceremonies. It was traditionally worn as a symbol of spiritual power and protection. It helps connect self to soul through the sense of longing. It has been said the path of the soul is also the path of the fool, the path of transparency. Thomas Moore puts it well:

> As we become transparent, revealed for exactly who we are and not who we wish to be, then the mystery of human life as a whole glistens momentarily in a flash of incarnation. Spirituality emanates from the ordinariness of this human life made transparent by lifelong tending to its nature and fate.[33]

This is no easy feat. It is not a matter of wishing it to be, but of allowing and letting go. This process is not something that we can make happen, but is something that happens to us, when we are ready. Moore continues:

> The path of the soul will not allow concealment of the shadow without unfortunate consequences.... Then your soul, cared for in courage, will be so solid, so weathered and mysterious, that divinity will emanate from your very being. You will have the spiritual radiance of the holy fool who has dared to live life as it presents itself and to unfold personality with heavy yet creative doses of imperfection.[34]

In the Tarot, the fool's journey is a metaphor for the innocent faith associated with the hard and difficult journey toward soul connection.

Native North Americans encouraged Contrary or Reverse Warrior behavior. Contraries did the opposite of normal social convention, including inverse speech, with yes meaning no, and so on. They played a key role in society by helping people reflect on the absurdity of social norms. They were not tricksters or clowns playing a role; they were exposing the rituals of their community for closer observation. The imperfections and inconsistencies of relationships were played out for all to see. By being contrary, they helped their society see themselves as a whole.

Contraries often result from exposed soul fragments not able to integrate into the present moment. The pieces of disconnection were buried under an acceptance of dysfunction.

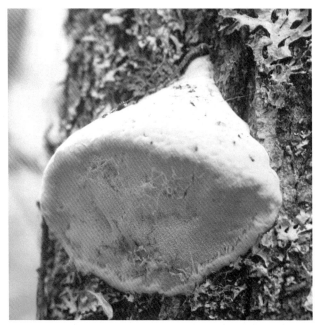

Diamond willow fungus (courtesy of Martin Osis)

Essence description

Diamond willow fungal essence helps us discover the true path of the soul. The essence helps us integrate soul fragments and helps support and nurture long-hidden parts of the soul, repressed by social convention from both present and past lives. The essence helps us emotionally recover more quickly from disappointment associated with expectations. It opens our eyes and hearts, and creates a deep longing for connection with our true nature.

It is useful to take this mushroom essence during what anthropologists call "vision quests." The Lakota word *hanblecheya* means "crying" or "lamenting." Fasting rituals, and soul-centered journeys of longing, are helped by diamond willow mushroom essence.

PREPARATION: This mushroom essence is produced by placing a small vial of rainwater with colloidal silver into a hole drilled in the mushroom fruiting body for an entire lunar cycle. It is best to start the cycle with the moon in the sign of Gemini or Aquarius.

CASE STUDY: Leonard was a gay aboriginal man, single, sixty-four years old. He came to me initially for advice involving a sexually transmitted disease. The infection was addressed with a combination of herbal and pharmaceutical protocols. He had moved to the city from his northern isolated community sixteen years ago and still felt estranged from nature and from his own people and culture. During one interview, he revealed he was physically and sexually abused as a young child and came from a family of addicts. He spent time as a young child in a residential school run by Roman Catholic priests and nuns. He was aware of the traditional use of diamond willow for smudging in sweat lodge ceremonies. I suggested he try diamond willow mushroom essence for a lunar cycle and keep a dream journal. He agreed, and by mid-cycle he began to dream about totem animals, particularly the bear and the moose.

On our next consultation, I suggested his visions were coming to assist his healing and reconnection with his people and culture. He understood and shed some tears. He took the same essence for a second lunar cycle, and it was profound. One night, his seven-year-old self came to him, damaged, abused, and frightened. I had suggested there was a scared young part of him that was in need of protection. He understood. I asked him his Cree name, and he whispered "Machk," meaning bear. I invited him to connect and speak with his younger self when the opportunity next came. It happened the next night.

In his dream state, he told his Machk that no one would hurt him anymore: he would protect him. Almost immediately, the energy pattern switched. He began to participate once more in indigenous sweat lodge ceremonies. Six months later he began to work with homeless aboriginal young people. He reowned his original name. A year later he presented me with a bear-claw necklace that I still treasure.

GRIFOLA · HEN OF THE WOODS · MAITAKE

(Grifola frondosa)

INDICATIONS: guilt, belief, integration, music, biomedicine, judgment, evidence-based medicine, harmony, dis-ease

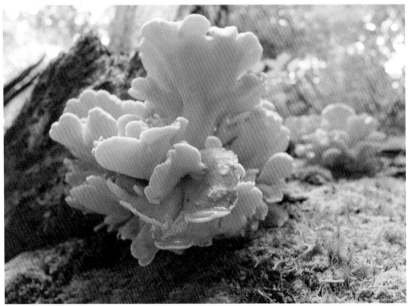

Hen of the woods (*Grifola frondosa* [Dickson] Gray) (courtesy of Alan McClelland)

Every disease is a musical problem. Every cure, a musical solution. The more rapid and complete the solution, the greater the musical talent of the doctor.

—NOVALIS

Let your meditation walk no further than pleasure, and even a little behind.

—FICINO

Around the world exists a vast variety of human healing modalities. In North America, the two main camps may be classified as biomedical (orthodox) or alternative. For a number of years, I have advocated an integrated health system that would provide health consumers the best of both worlds in the prevention and treatment of dis-ease. Because the issue is divisive, and based on belief systems and turf management, the two camps rarely cooperate. A great deal of effort is wasted on negativity and judgment.

The attitude of many allopathic doctors is the belief that everything can be explained scientifically or else it is not valid. In fact, the recent trend in biomedicine is evidence-based medicine, the use of mathematical equations to decide what course of drugs or surgical treatment works best for the majority of patients. For a critique of this limited approach to wellness, read Steve Hickey and Hilary Roberts's *Tarnished Gold: The Sickness of Evidence-Based Medicine.*

On the other hand, there are many people who believe all things natural are good and can do no harm. This is likewise an unproductive and dangerous position. Harmonious patterns are found throughout the universe. Women living together begin to harmonize their menstrual cycles. Professors and students show similar brain waves when thinking about things they recognize. Hearts lying beside each other in an operating room begin to beat in harmony once exposed to each other. Freud's Hungarian colleague Sándor Ferenczi suggested our body parts have their own "organ eroticism."[35] This suggests they don't simply work; they also enjoy themselves.

The word *disease* means "not having your elbows in a relaxed position." Ease is from the Latin *ansatus,* meaning "having handles," or "elbows akimbo," a relaxed position. *Dis-ease* means "no elbows," "no elbow room." Ease is a form of pleasure, dis-ease is a loss of pleasure. Disharmony is chaos. Edward Bach wrote, "Disease is, in essence, the result of conflict between Soul and Mind ... and will never be eradicated except by spiritual and mental effort."[36]

Essence description

Grifola mushroom essence helps us to appreciate different perspectives on health and healing. It helps individuals decide for themselves the model of wellness that best suits their own belief system, without guilt or remorse.

Grifola mushroom essence may help individuals looking to gain balance and perspectives on the wildly conflicting opinions offered by members of various healing professions. It helps provide deeper insights into our own health condition and reconnection with our own self-healing powers.

Grifola mushroom essence helps us understand the need to be responsible for our ease by asking various parts of the body if they are relaxed. Tension held in various organs requires attention. Ask the liver, for example, "Am I doing something that is making you depressed? Where is your body not pleasurable?" Moore suggests:

> We could imagine disease as not just a physical phenomenon but as a condition of the person and world, as the failure of the body to find its pleasure. Pleasure does not necessarily refer to the gratification of the senses or the frenzied pursuit of new experiences, possessions, or entertainments. We might notice dreams that occur at the time of an illness. We could tone down the masculine heroics in the modern practice of medicine and allow some freedom of imagination.[37]

Wellness is not simply the absence of disease, but is a state of connection with soul.

PREPARATION: Grifola mushroom essence is produced with rainwater in a crystal bowl in two parts. One preparation is done during the new moon, and another during the waning of the moon. The two waters and brandy are combined in equal parts.

CASE STUDY: Sonia was a forty-four-year-old woman, working as a registered nurse, married with two children. She had been recently diagnosed with cervical cancer and was referred to a surgeon and oncologist. She came to my clinic wanting to know if there were natural alternatives to a hysterectomy or radiation therapy. We discussed her various options, but it was obvious she was uncertain which way to go. I suggested she take Grifola mushroom essence for one lunar cycle to assist her process.

She returned exactly four weeks later and told me about a dream she experienced. She was lying in her bath, and slowly a round-faced moon emerged from her genital area. It smiled at her, opened its mouth, and swallowed itself. She awoke, shaking all over.

The next day, she booked herself for a cervical cone biopsy. The results showed cancer in stage 1A1 and confirmation that the human papilloma virus (HPV) was involved. Together, we then developed a protocol using herbal and homeopathic thuja and calendula. Three months later, there was no sign of cervical dysplasia.

SPLIT GILL

(Schizophyllum commune)

INDICATIONS: chronic fatigue, circadian rhythm, insomnia, pineal gland, sin, sex

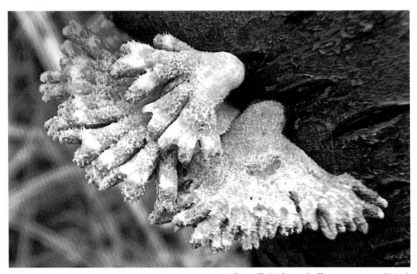

Split gill (*Schizophyllum commune* Fries)

Sexuality is one of the ways that we become enlightened,
actually, because it leads us to self-knowledge.

—ALICE WALKER

Split gill is a fairly common tiny mushroom. Research has found split gill has twenty-eight thousand different ways in which it can engage in sex. Even the Kama Sutra falls far short of this astounding number of reproductive opportunities. Mushroom extracts have been researched in Japan for the treatment of chronic fatigue syndrome.

The top side is somewhat hairy or furry and is usually white to brown-white. The mandala-like underside produces numerous spores, light brown in nature. Brown is sometimes associated with lack of awareness,[1] according to Graves. But this mushroom is far from unaware. The split gills represent polarity and opposites. The hairy top is related to extreme sensitivity on the higher plane, while the wavy, frazzled underneath of the fruiting body represents stress, irritation, and nervous excitability.

When our planet is viewed from space at night, numerous urban centers are fully illuminated. For our pineal gland to produce melatonin for sound restful sleep, full darkness is necessary. Sleep is the time when the immune system becomes restored and initiates repairs. The liver cleanses efficiently, and the entire system relaxes and regenerates. Chronic inflammation subsides, and the dream state brings awareness to a plethora of subconscious messages.

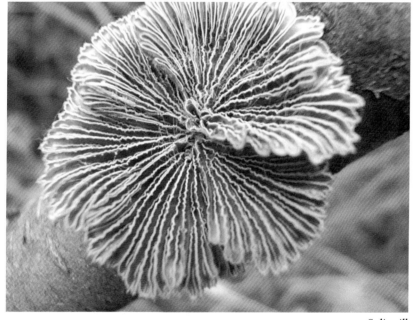

Split gill

Essence description

Split gill mushroom essence is related to the restoration of our circadian rhythm in modern life. It combines well with chaga mushroom essence for health of the pineal gland and production of melatonin.

Many individuals, upon taking this mushroom essence, will experience erotic or sexually themed dreams that may frighten, excite, or disturb. In most cases, this is to be expected and is usually temporary.

Split gill mushroom essence may help dissipate the angst, guilt, and self-reprimand associated with early childhood sexual issues. Children raised in strict fundamentalist families will find the opportunity as mature adults to reexamine their patterns and beliefs equating sex and sin.

In fact, the essence may help us become more comfortable with sexuality in general, and may be useful for transgendered, gay, lesbian, and other individuals seeking to define or find themselves through individual sexual expression. For younger people, it may help them connect, discover, or begin to understand their own sexual orientation. Split gill essence may help people accept various phases of sexual life associated with aging, changing levels of sexual frequency, and increased awareness of issues around intimacy.

It may also help those individuals who engage in or have suffered from self-injury in early exploration of their sexual identity. Spirituality and sexuality are intertwined and spiral as an expression of creativity and abundance. This helps create soul growth and prosperity on many levels.

PREPARATION: Split gill essence is produced by placing the fruiting body on rainwater, in a crystal bowl, under a moon influenced by Scorpio or Gemini.

CASE STUDY: Tom was a seventeen-year-old student raised in a family practicing the Jehovah's Witness religion. He came to my office with his parents, who were concerned about his ongoing insomnia, exhaustion, and nervous fatigue. He complained he was unable to concentrate on studies and was lethargic and stressed. Sleep medications were not working. I asked the parents if I could have a few moments alone with their son. They reluctantly consented and I quickly shifted the conversation to sexual orientation. He was very defensive, so I asked if he had a girlfriend or went on dates. He looked down and whispered "no." I suggested he take split gill mushroom essence for twenty-eight days and keep a dream journal.

He thought his parents would disapprove, so I recommended a nervine and adaptogenic herbal formula, into which I put 50 drops of essence in a 100-milliliter tincture blend. He took this at a dose of 30 drops twice daily for the next month. He returned a month later, with his parents, who sat outside in the waiting room, again at his request. He looked much more relaxed, and reported he was sleeping better. He confided that he had experienced very erotic and sexual dreams, and had a wet dream one night. He had been concerned that he was gay, as before this, he had not really thought of girls. I asked him what he wanted to do. He replied, "I can hardly wait for college, so I can start my own life."

LUMINESCENT PANELLUS
(Panellus stipticus)

INDICATIONS: body language, introversion, self-image, stuttering, stage fright, communication, subconscious, nonverbal, writing

Panellus means "small torch," in reference to its bioluminescence.

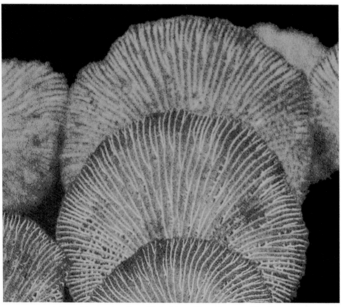

Luminescent Panellus (*Panellus stipticus* [Bulliard] Karsten)
(courtesy of Taylor F. Lockwood)

I'd stand in the shadows of your heart and tell
you I'm not afraid of your dark.
—ANDREA GIBSON

As far as we can discern, the sole purpose of human existence
is to kindle a light in the darkness of mere being.
—CARL JUNG

Luminescent Panellus emits light when discharging spores, but this stops when it is dried. If remoistened, even after six months, the fruiting body again becomes luminous. European and North American forms are morphologically indistinguishable, but the Old World mushroom does not glow green and does not possess myco-luminescence. Several species of mushroom, including species in genera *Armillaria, Pleurotus, Omphalina,* and *Mycena,* glow with a green color in the mycelium or fruiting body, or both. There are now over sixty known *Mycena* species on the planet with this unusual but fascinating characteristic.

Why do they glow? No one is really sure, but a few hypotheses include attraction of spore-bearing insects or a possible side-effect of lignin consumption. The energy associated with light production and the evolutionary pathways leading to this unique mushroom expression are most interesting. Could there be a more spiritual connection, a more esoteric answer to this question? Mushrooms are more closely related, in evolutionary terms, to animals and humans than plants. If the light is used for communication, what is it saying? Is it repelling enemies or attracting friends? Perhaps it's a bit of both.

Essence description

Luminescent Panellus mushroom essence is related to subconscious and nonverbal communication skills. Body language, for example, will reveal various emotions that are held inside but not expressed. The mushroom essence helps us observe body language in others and become aware of the message they express through their posture and other nonverbal communication. Human communication is 20 percent verbal and 80 percent nonverbal.

There are many issues related to human communication. Stuttering, for example, is an expression of poor self-image; a veil that helps hide our true self from others. Stuttering may represent a blocked soul mission. Other manifestations may be chronic sore throat, tongue sores, or dental and gum problems.

Open arms express welcome, and crossed or closed arms represent guardedness, fending off attack, or unwelcome annoyance. It may represent a stance against opposition.

It is no coincidence the color green is expressed during myco-luminescence. This is the color of the plant kingdom, the expression of chlorophyll and the ability to create energy from the sun. Mushrooms rely on plants for sugar and in exchange provide protection, nutrients, and water to their floral friends. Green is calming and cooling in nature and relates to the lung and heart chakra. Green is the middle color of the rainbow. It is the midpoint between dark and light.

Luminescent Panellus is about coming out, about speaking our truth and standing up for our understanding of reality. The essence supports those who suffer stage fright or are afraid to write, produce, or share their vision with others. One of our most healing moments in life is telling our story to others. And the greatest gift to anyone is to *really* hear their story. Poetry, both written and read, is another pathway to soul connection. This mushroom essence is excellent for modern-day bards. It is an essence for the introvert, who has something to contribute, especially around issues involving nature, human nature, ecology, and the environment.

It is more than passive resistance; it is a voice that speaks for the great underworld of deep wisdom and understanding. Putting vision into words, or vice versa, is greatly eased with the use of luminescent Panellus mushroom essence.

PREPARATION: The mushroom essence is produced from biolumines-cent fruiting bodies indoors in complete darkness, or outside during one of three nights around the new moon. This essence may be produced, if necessary, from fruiting bodies grown indoors. When the moon is in Gemini is the ideal time for preparation. Gently set the fruiting bodies on top of rainwater in a crystal bowl for at least four hours.

CASE STUDY: George was a twenty-six-year-old man, finishing a master's degree in philosophy. He had recently been accepted at Oxford University to complete his PhD. He came to my clinic to see if I could help with his stuttering. I expressed interest in his subject of interest and he sent me a copy of one of his early papers. His academic and writing skills were exceptional, but they lacked a certain passion or emotional "juice."

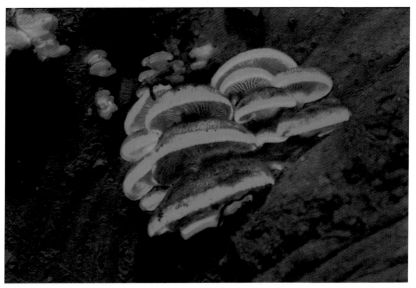

Luminescent Panellus (courtesy of Keith Garrett)

We met again, and he began with a lunar cycle of the mushroom essence. I requested that he keep a dream journal. He returned at the end of the cycle and was very pleased and relieved. His stuttering, worse in public, had improved about "70 percent," in his own words. What was really interesting was the quality of writing in his dream journal. The first week to ten days were rather mundane, in both content and style. But in the following weeks, it was as if a portal of conscious awareness had opened. It was as if he had found his true voice. He confided that he was in the middle of his master's thesis and was concerned this breakthrough would affect his writing style. I reassured him that it was only bound to improve. Six months later, he came to thank me and say good-bye before flying to England. He defended his dissertation without any significant stuttering. His public stuttering phase was, by and large, over.

HONEY MUSHROOM

(Armillaria solidipes and related species*)*

INDICATIONS: elder wisdom, midlife crisis, projection, gall bladder, flexibility, friendship

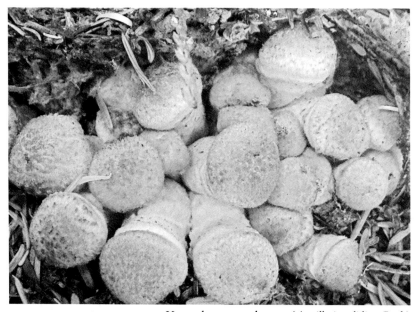

Young honey mushroom (*Armillaria solidipes* Peck)

No man can taste the fruits of autumn while he is
delighting his scent with the flowers of spring.
—SAMUEL JOHNSON

Destiny has summoned the hero and transferred his spiritual center
of gravity from within the pale of his society to a zone unknown.
—JOSEPH CAMPBELL

Honey mushroom is the largest organism on earth. One individual mycelium community growing in Oregon is 2,400 acres in size and over two thousand years old. It would be fair to say a great deal of ancient wisdom is associated with this particular mushroom.

Brown, white, and yellow coloration are found in both young and old honey mushrooms. Yellow is the color of youth, joy, and radiance. It is related to the liver and gall bladder, and in turn, the emotions of repressed anger.

Honey mushrooms appear when there is a turn of seasons, when the summer warmth turns to autumn chill. It is a signal for the fruiting bodies to complete their destiny of reproduction. In humans this is also observed. In the fall or middle age of people, there is often a reexamination of priorities and a reassessment of life plans. In some cases, the ego has become too hardened and inflexible, and the soul awaits the opportunity to create a trauma or a moment of growth. In the perpetually adolescent male, this can lead to a midlife crisis with the clichéd red sports car and a younger second or third "trophy" wife. In the menopausal crone, this time can lead to deep introspection and reexamination of previous life decisions.

Society is not supportive of midlife change and interferes in three ways. It encourages people not to change, it helps people stay the same, and it alienates those who disrupt any norms. In reality, a midlife crisis is a midlife transformation. It is a time to reconnect, simplify, and change. It is the time of soul reconnection.

Essence description

Honey mushroom essence can be most useful when the search for perpetual or regained youth, or the feeling life is passing too quickly, can lead to impetuous action. The desire to return to adolescence is, of course, fraught with emotional danger. It will often lead us back to square one, in the search for self-awareness or soul development. Women will desire a way to shift from caretaker and mothering to exploring their own growth potential and self-actualization. This can be a good thing. Edward C. Whitmont notes:

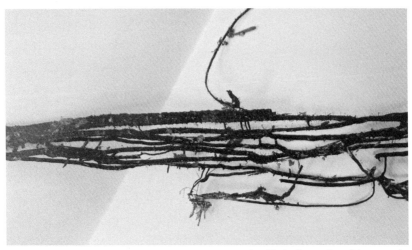

Armillaria shoestring rhizomorphs

A projection invariably blurs our own view of the other person … and interferes with our capacity to see objectively and relate humanly. Imagine an automobile driver who, unknowingly, wears spectacles of red glass. He would find it difficult to tell the difference between red, yellow, or green traffic lights, and he would be in constant danger of an accident. It is of no help to him that some, or for that matter, even most of the lights he perceives as red really happen to be red. The danger to him comes from the inability to differentiate and separate, which his "red projection" imposes on him. Where a shadow projection occurs we are not able to differentiate between the actuality of the other person and our own complexes.[2]

Couples going through this phase together will benefit from honey essence in that the issues are similar and addressed by internal acknowledgment of the autumn of life. Remember, this is not winter, but autumn, a season rich in transition and beauty. It is the time of harvest and gathering of the fruits of labor.

It is the time of life when accumulated wisdom can be freely shared with others in our community. Elders provide an important element of mentoring that has been lost in modern North American life, with its socially accepted overemphasis on nursing homes, extended care facilities, and inevitable separation from loved ones.

Honey mushroom mycelia are myco-luminescent, but the fruiting bodies are not. This also is interesting, as the reproductive part sees no need to shine upon itself, but appears when needed. The organism itself shines within and without. Some of our teachers, our wise elders, are like that. They appear when they are needed.

Honey mushroom essence helps us recognize the gift of friendship around us and openly thank friends for their contributions to our lives. Many will be unaware of their impact and will feel blessed by our recognition.

PREPARATION: This mushroom essence is produced from both fruiting bodies and rhizomorphs during the waning of the moon, using rainwater and brandy. The large branching rhizomorphs are quite distinct, often called shoestrings. Preparation under the lunar influence of Capricorn or Sagittarius is ideal.

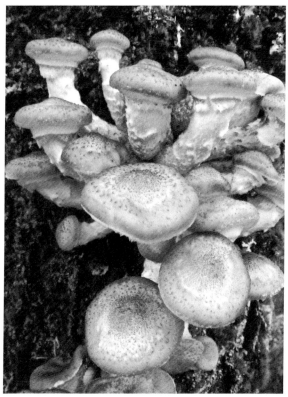

Honey mushrooms

CASE STUDY: An older couple, he fifty-eight and she fifty-six, married for thirty-five years, came to my clinical practice at the recommendation of their psychologist, a good friend of mine. They wanted help with a lack of communication in their relationship. They both expressed the feeling they were growing apart. She was fully into menopause. He was semiretired. They were empty-nesters, with their children and grandchildren in another city. He wanted to travel; she wanted to garden. He was starting to cross off his bucket list, and she wanted to explore inner growth and goddess work.

I recommended honey mushroom essence for each of them and suggested they keep a dream journal as well. A lunar cycle later, they returned, and the difference in demeanor was obvious. It was as if they had fallen in love again. They found that by sharing their journal writing, there were a number of shared concerns and aspirations that reignited the reason for their initial attraction as soul mates. As they were leaving, he turned to me and said, "I guess I don't have to buy that red convertible after all."

SHIITAKE
(Lentinula edodes)

INDICATIONS: control, racism, cultural awareness, fear, judgment, shadow work, adoption, abandonment, antibiotics

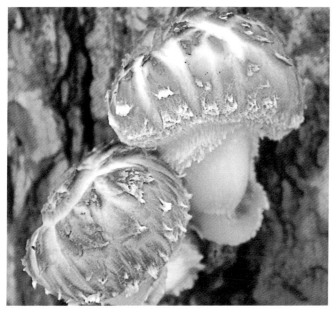

Shiitake (*Lentinula edodes* [Berkeley] Pegler)

Thinking is difficult; that's why most people judge.
—CARL JUNG

*Preservation of one's own culture does not require
contempt or disrespect for other cultures.*
—CESAR CHAVEZ

*Darkness cannot drive out darkness; only light can do that.
Hate cannot drive out hate; only love can do that.*
—MARTIN LUTHER KING JR.

Lent- means "pliable" or "supple," and *-inus* means "resembling." *Edodes* means "edible." *Shiitake* refers to its relationship with a species of oak. When we look closely at young shiitake fruiting bodies, a noticeable pink color moving toward violet will be observed. Pink is the color of vulnerability, love, and tenderness. Light purple represents spirituality, oneness, and a sense of abundance.

Taken in this context, the mushroom essence may be useful in a number of ways. Individuals who have been abandoned, adopted, or raised in a culture that differs from their genetic roots will find the essence helpful in adjusting to or accepting their new family and home. This may be helpful at any stage or age of life.

Multiculturalism can add to the variety and spice of a community, but it may also create tension, hostility, and resentment. One of the difficulties surrounding racism is our inability to tolerate any challenge to our racial reality. We either shut down or we strike out in an attempt to block out any reflection of our discomfort.

Essence description

Shiitake mushroom essence helps us develop a deeper understanding of culture. Culture shock, adjustment, and awareness play key roles in helping us understand other human beings and their worldview.

When someone is not feeling comfortable because they are a visible minority, shiitake mushroom essence may give additional support and comfort. Shiitake essence helps us embrace our own culture and revel in its uniqueness and vitality, but also learn to love and accept other cultures and people for their generosity and sharing. Travelers to new countries will find this essence useful in helping to restrain judgment and criticism of their new surroundings. It will help sharpen awareness of cultural mores and prevent inadvertent faux pas by increasing sensitivity to their surroundings.

Social and cultural interactions stir up the shadow side of the collective unconscious. In fact, the primal root of social, racial, and national bias and discrimination is our own internal split or struggle. Jung says it best: "Recognition of the shadow … leads to the modesty we need in order to acknowledge imperfection. And it is just this conscious recognition and consideration that are needed wherever a human relationship is to be established."[3]

The shadow is not eliminated, but when we cannot see it, we should be aware of the fact that we cannot see it. Shiitake essence helps us understand that having prejudice is not the problem; the problem is that we blindly assume we do not have any.

Awareness of unconscious racism is enhanced. Joachim-Ernst Berendt writes:

> If therefore Western philosophy's love of wisdom and truth primarily involves separating, judging, and criticizing, then it is a philosophy of seeing. Separation of the world into observer and observed, subject and object, which is the precondition for criticism, creates distance and remoteness.[4]

At the basis of all judgment is fear. When we operate from a place of fear, we are more likely to be reactive and less observant. We want to control the situation rather than let things unfold. Shiitake mushroom essence enhances our ability to relax and let go in new environments and cultures.

Another aspect of shiitake relates to how we view our body. Moore writes:

> We might imagine much of our current disease as the body asserting itself in a context of cultural numbing. The stomach takes no pleasure in frozen and powdered foods. The back of the neck complains about polyester. The feet die of boredom for lack of walking in interesting places. The brain is depressed to find itself described as a computer, and the heart surely doesn't enjoy being treated as a pump. There isn't much opportunity to exercise the spleen these days, and the liver is no longer the seat of passion. All these noble, richly poetic organs, teeming with meaning and power, have been made into functions. We are perhaps the only culture to regard the body with such poverty of imagination.[5]

Shiitake mushroom essence may help in another way. Billions, maybe trillions, of various intestinal bacteria work in concert with us to provide optimal health and well-being. Various drugs, including antibiotics ("anti-life"), destroy and disrupt this carefully balanced population of diverse living beings. Taking shiitake mushroom essence for a lunar cycle may energetically create more ideal conditions for intestinal floral growth to flourish. Fermented foods, created by various members of the kingdom Fungi, help reestablish healthy intestinal balance.

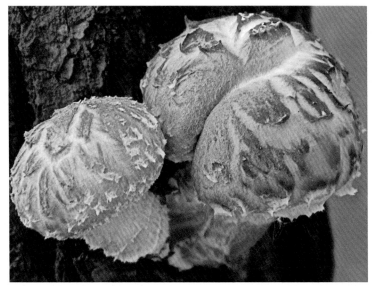

Shiitake mushrooms

PREPARATION: This mushroom essence is produced from shiitake freshly sliced with a ceramic knife, layered on top of rainwater in a crystal bowl. This is ideally done on the night of the full moon, but it's not absolutely critical. Several factors suggest that a moon full in an air sign might be best, but further trials will be necessary to confirm this hypothesis. The lunar influence of Libra and Aquarius may be most useful, or perhaps Sagittarius, if the issue involves travel.

CASE STUDY: Frank was a fifty-eight-year-old man, recently divorced. His six children were all over the world, getting on with their own lives. He was the manager of a coffee franchise, where 80 percent of his staff were immigrants earning minimum wage. He came to me initially for an enlarged prostate (benign prostatic hyperplasia), and we were quite successful in reducing the size and frequency of his night-time urinations with the help of medicinal mushrooms.

It was obvious in our first meeting that he was worried, frustrated, and concerned about other issues. He admitted his job of managing immigrant workers was difficult; he felt they did not like him. I asked him if he liked his workers. He hesitated and said, "They are alright for … people." I suggested to him racism was an all too familiar issue, which he quickly and vehemently denied. I let it sit for a moment and suggested he try shiitake mushroom essence for a month. He quickly agreed, probably to get out of the uncomfortable seat in which I had placed him.

He returned in a few weeks, looked sheepish and guilty. He had taken the shiitake mushroom essence drops as suggested and immediately became aware of a different vibration at work. He began to feel like an outsider in his own business and initially wanted to hide himself in his small windowless office. As the weeks went on, he began to notice a change within himself. He began to acknowledge to himself that he was indeed racist, and remembered his father was a horribly racist individual.

He confided to me that his youngest daughter had married an immigrant. He found himself unable to attend his own daughter's wedding, which contributed to the breakup of his own marriage. He was overcome with this realization, and the extreme emotions associated with his racial prejudice. Over the next several months, he continued taking shiitake and a combination of other mushroom essences, including varnish conk, maze gill, and Oregon white truffle. He struggled at times, but gradually he became thankful for these new insights. He began to interact in a more respectful manner with his staff. He experienced a Scrooge-like readjustment of his prejudice. During our final appointment, he confided to me that he had phoned his daughter and asked her forgiveness. They met the next day; they cried and reconciled. The healing had begun.

NOTE: Astrology and mycology have some interesting correspondences. One study conducted by Michael Barreto was a year-long investigation in 2006 and 2007 into shiitake inoculation, cultivation, and lunar cycles. The signs of the zodiac were divided into the four elements— earth, water, air, and fire. Those involved in making the substrate blocks were not aware of the double-blind procedure. The greatest mushroom yields were obtained when shiitake inoculation occurred with the moon in fire and air signs. The highest yields were under the influence of air signs and lowest on earth sign days.[6]

GREEN DEATH CAP

(Amanita phalloides)

INDICATIONS: repetition, defensiveness, depression, repression, will, dreams, indoctrination, sorrow, feeling, dogs, earthquakes, diamonds

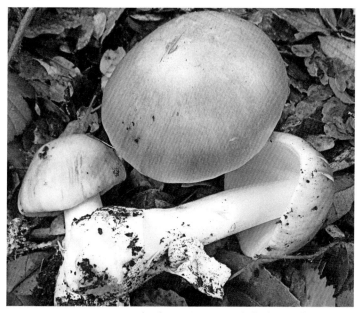

Green death cap (*Amanita phalloides* [Vaillant] Link)

This above all; to thine own self be true.
—SHAKESPEARE, HAMLET *1.3*

The authentic self is the soul made visible.
—SARAH BAN BREATHNACH

We have all been deeply indoctrinated since childhood about sense of self, learned largely from observing the behavior of our mother and father. Mother, of course, represents our natural life, and any distortion or issues of earthly pleasure can later manifest into emotional and mental difficulties. Father represents order, and breaking away from his belief system can feel like dread or create a paralysis of will.

The absence of either parent in a young child's life will shape the way the child interprets his or her sense of self. We are a copy of our parents' life experience, and the grooves in our brain are similar to the well-rutted channels on an old phonographic record. That is, behaviors that are repeated and rewarded, even if dysfunctional, create an automatic response of behavior.

The analogy of a scratchy old analog recording and a new digital composition is worth exploring. Analog signals are represented by a continuous stream of data and involve physical alteration of this continuous signal. Before digital technology, analog signal processing was our only method to manipulate a signal. A digital representation expresses pressure waveforms as a sequence of symbols, usually binary numbers. Digital represents today, and analog is a reminder of yesterday. How many people are ignoring the symbols presented to us on a day-to-day basis, and instead move on the same groove day after day, year after year?

Sound in mind, sound in body. We have all heard this expression, but what does it really mean? It is often invoked when we write our will, a legal expression of our wishes for distribution of our earthly possessions when we die. Thinking is a consciously willed act. But feelings happen as moods, and thoughts occur, regardless of our conscious will. Whitmont writes, "Hence it is an error to assume that we can control our thoughts, not to mention our feelings, simply by resolving to do so.… We cannot choose to have thoughts or feelings that will not come, nor can we choose not to have those that do."[7] We can channel these thoughts and feelings into acceptable form by conscious confrontation, but not by avoidance. Avoidance is a repressed state that will manifest into shadow that, unowned, may lead to repression or depression and our emotional downfall. Our liver is associated with depression and the nature of will. Twentyman writes:

> [Depression] is the state which arises when the will is paralyzed to a greater or lesser extent.… We cannot think the future or intellectually plan it, we will it. Paralysis of the will therefore is one way for describing that state in which we experience being cut off from the future and thrown one-sidedly upon the past. If we can relate only to the past and to the inevitable continuation of the past which

mechanism implies and which intellectual thought can alone grasp and accept, we cannot escape overwhelming guilt and despair.

One can see in some cases that deep sorrow, which is not psychically digested and metamorphosed into wisdom, and sinks down into the liver. It becomes not transformed but buried and then may become later the basis of endogenous depression.[8]

The Bedouin will say to a loved one, "I give you my liver." Not the heart, as we romanticize in Western culture, but the organ system associated with repressed emotions and depressed manifestations. Death cap mushroom is extremely toxic, and if ingested will very likely cause kidney and liver failure and death. It combines very well with cinnabar and birch polypore mushroom essence.

Essence description

My logical left-brain told me death cap was about death and rebirth. I wanted this to be so, and when I prepared the mushroom essence, I anticipated a revelatory journey in that direction. Much to my surprise, the essence is about our sense of self. When we are confronted on our values and personal habits, we become defensive, as if the extinction of ourselves is at stake. Our egos impede self-growth and attempt to stop the process of soul integration. This can lead to issues involving the liver and depression.

Indeed, the essence relates to our deepest relationship with self, and the continual brainwashing of our own minds. Death cap mushroom essence helps us recognize and challenge our early patterns of socialization and find the path to more conscious awareness. It is about being true to self, and about a more authentic path to soul connection.

Dreams may include dogs, body parts, cancer, earthquakes, pursuits, and family. The appearance of diamonds as an instrument of healing may be present. Jung noted that even the diamond body of an enduring self can be formed. The diamond body comes from lead in water, a cold, heavy metal, according to Chinese yoga. From the body (*muladhara*) or the water center (*svadhisthana*), alchemy produces god or the diamond body. Jung suggests in *Dream Analysis* that "the concept of the diamond body is really identical with the idea of the subtle body."[9]

What earthquake is taking place internally? What pressures are keeping us from soul connection? It helps us recognize our groove may simply be a rut, and increased awareness and self-observation will assist the necessary transition to soul work.

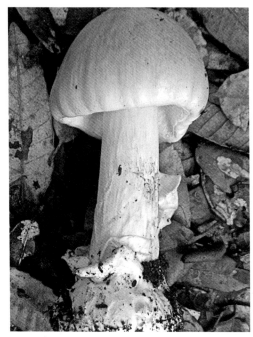

Green death cap

PREPARATION: Death cap mushroom essence is prepared by filling inverted caps with rainwater under a full moon. This is combined with equal parts of brandy the next morning. Because this essence is about being true to self, it is best prepared under the moon in your own personal sun sign.

CAUTION: The toxin phalloidin is not water soluble, but can cause transdermal poisoning. Due to the poisonous nature of this mushroom, it is advised you either purchase this mushroom essence or prepare it for your own use by placing a dropper bottle containing equal parts rainwater and brandy on top of the photograph in this book for twenty-four hours.

CASE STUDY: Wendy was a twenty-six-year-old bank clerk with a steady boyfriend. She came to me because she was unable to achieve orgasm. She enjoyed sex, due to the feeling of intimacy, but was left feeling unsatisfied. She had left home when she was eighteen and had not spoken to either of her parents for seven years. She blamed them for her unhappy childhood. I suggested she take green death cap mushroom essence for a lunar cycle and write in a dream journal. She agreed.

That month, she had a recurring dream in which she had lost a diamond and was searching for it. The constant nightly pursuits were exhausting her. She was being attacked by dogs that were tearing off her legs and arms. I asked her if she would like to marry, and she responded that she was patiently waiting for her boyfriend to pop the question. I suggested that because it was a leap year, women can ask men to marry them on February 29. This was only three weeks away. She came back a month later with a diamond ring on her finger, a big smile on her face, and the revelation that she had, at last, achieved climax during sex. She initiated a reunion with her parents, who attended her wedding about a year later, at the beginning of her Saturn return.

SHAGGY MANE

(Coprinus comatus)

INDICATIONS: control, jealousy, masculinity, writer's block, occupation, pornography, frustration, sexism, professional sports

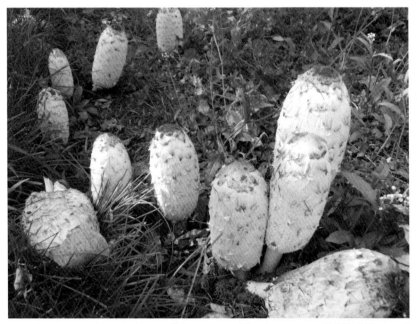

Shaggy mane (*Coprinus comatus* [Müller] Persoon)

The male-dominant agenda is so fragile that
any competitor is felt as a deadly foe.

—TERENCE MCKENNA

I am tired, beloved, of chafing my heart against the want of you;
Of squeezing it into little ink drops, and posting it.
And I scald alone, here, under the fire of the great moon.

—AMY LOWELL

Shaggy mane fruiting body self-destructs in order to regenerate. This process, known as deliquescence, equates to the proverbial disappearing act.

The mushroom fruiting bodies pop up in massive amounts and overrun and monopolize others. In many ways, shaggy mane is the soldier, policeman, or Klingon of the kingdom Fungi. The process requires control and yet possession of perfect timing. Shaggy mane is a very powerful mushroom. The soft fruiting body exerts enough hydraulic pressure to break through thick concrete slabs.

Early in life, young boys are taught to endure pain, never cry or complain but possess a stiff upper lip and be strong. This early belief system can be devastating and result in long-term repercussions for today's adult male. It will often require several bouts of severe trauma and ego defeat to trigger soul encounter. Due to today's increased equality of the sexes, and the dualistic role of protector and sensitive individual, many modern males find it difficult to access their true feelings.

Shaggy mane mushroom essence is especially useful for those who cannot easily answer this question: "What is it that you really would like to do with your life?" Many times, in order to please family, a partner, a boss, or the community, men will avoid discussions about how they feel. They may have a difficult time connecting with others and then expressing how they truly feel. Frustration, denial, and various methods of avoidance are the result of not knowing how to acknowledge their true masculine nature, wants, and desires.

When confronted with this situation, the male will often "disappear," at least on the mental and emotional level. If the tension becomes too much, and there is no release of pent-up angst, they may leave physically as well. Machismo attitudes are often associated with fear and the need for control, or at least playing the role of being in control.

Essence description

Shaggy mane mushroom essence represents the quintessential male, following the model of John Wayne and other strong, silent archetypes of stage and screen. The essence may help males move beyond the superficiality found in parts of modern North American life. Typical recreational patterns such as watching the game, hunting, fishing, drinking beer, and telling sexist jokes may quickly lose their appeal while taking the mushroom essence.

Modern Western society worships professional sports and athletes in a manner reminiscent of the Roman gladiators. Armchair quarterbacks live vicariously through ritualistic rote, right down to purchasing and consuming the very alcoholic beverages advertised during intermission. Cybersex and online pornography addiction may replace spiritually connected lovemaking in some individuals. Pornography, for men, leads to objectification of women, endorsing or condoning the industry, isolation, and confusion around real women.

Shallow responses begin to ring hollow, and longtime relationships with friends can be strained by the emotional roller coaster of soul reconnection. When taking shaggy mane mushroom essence, the shock to the psyche can be jarring. Attention is important.

Shaggy mane mushroom essence may help prepare women desiring a career in traditional male occupations. The construction trades, in particular, can be emotionally and mentally challenging for women unaccustomed to macho male behavior. Striving to become "one of the guys" is a discredit to everyone involved, as women possess special gifts of intuition and imagination that can be brought to the workplace.

This mushroom essence is useful for those who are critical of other occupations. Tradespeople often disparage the "suits" and "white collars," who in turn are often condescending toward individuals who enjoy physical labor. A healthy balance of the physical and mental planes is necessary to live without judgment or jealousy. Soul purpose is about much more than occupation. It is about embarking on a life journey of self-discovery, finding our true vocation, and creating a truly full life.

Shaggy mane may be a useful remedy for writer's block, that painful moment at the keyboard, staring at a blank screen. A few drops held under the tongue can be inspiring, and in some cases, catalytic or cathartic. Writer's block is well known to authors. It is the constriction or paralysis of attaching words to ideas and relates to overthinking and overanalyzing sentence form and structure. Shaggy mane mushroom essence helps trigger free flow with a direct conduit from the heart to the page. Try it and see! It also works in a similar manner for artists of any modality, from painters to sculptors to weavers and others.

At the root of this issue is a simple need to acknowledge our feelings and act on them. Shaggy mane mushroom essence helps bring awareness and harmony to our sense of self and, in turn, reconnection with soul. It combines well with dog stinkhorn for issues specifically around masculinity.

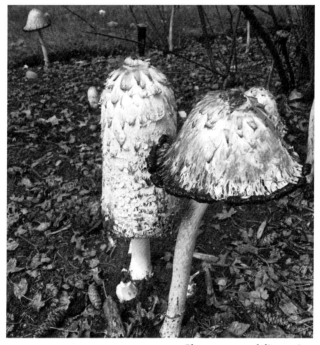

Shaggy mane deliquescing

PREPARATION: The mushroom essence is produced overnight by covering the surface of rainwater in a crystal bowl with the "ink," or deliquescence, produced by mature fruiting bodies. The particular phase of the lunar cycle is less critical for this essence.

CASE STUDY: Neil was a twenty-nine-year-old bartender and self-admitted jock who loved watching sports on television and hanging out with his buds. He came to see me for genital herpes. He owned up to being a bit of a hound dog when it came to seducing young women. In fact, he noted with a sense of pride, he was nearly up to his "century conquest." I asked him if he was feeling fulfilled in life, and he responded that his job and life were great. He admitted enjoying pornography and said he had several sexual partners who enjoyed watching it with him. In further conversation he revealed enjoying digital sex more than his human encounters. "There is no commitment and no awkward avoidance," he told me. I asked him if he had ever cried, to which he responded, "Not since I was a young boy." I suggested he take shaggy mane mushroom essence for twenty-eight days and note any dreams or differences in how he perceived himself and others. I also asked him to keep a journal.

He came back two months later and was most distraught. He had met a girl at the bar and was instantly smitten with her. He asked her for a date, and she turned him down. He admitted he could not get her out of his mind and could think of nothing else. He even stopped watching porn as it started to bore him. I suggested he take shaggy mane and giant puffball mushroom essences together for one more lunar cycle.

He came back to me about ten days later, asking my advice. He had asked the same young woman out again, and she told him that she was looking for "a real man," not a macho man. This threw him for a loop, as he had no idea what she meant. I suggested to him that one of the problems with modern North American life was the abundance of adolescent adults and the near absence of mature adults. I suggested he read the book *Fire in the Belly: On Being a Man,* by Sam Keen, and get back to me in a month.

The emotional shift, upon his next visit, was astounding. He had read the book and continued taking the shaggy mane and giant puffball mushroom essences for that month. I did not see him for over half a year. On his last visit, he thanked me for helping him begin to understand what it means to be a real man. He had quit his job, but did not get the girl. We hugged, and he cried. And I smiled.

OYSTER

(Pleurotus populinus)

INDICATIONS: acceptance, aloofness, arrogance, burning, conceit, deceit, dreams, gratefulness, humility, pride, shadow work, projection, divorce, awareness, attention

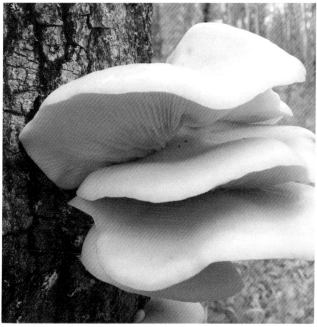

Oyster (*Pleurotus populinus* O. Hilber & O. K. Miller)

*And the Devil did grin, for his darling sin
Is pride that apes humility.*

—SAMUEL TAYLOR COLERIDGE, *THE DEVIL'S THOUGHTS*

*Through pride we are ever deceiving ourselves. But deep
down below the surface of the average conscience a still,
small voice says to us, something is out of tune.*

—CARL JUNG

Arrogance is a creature. It does not have senses. It has only a sharp tongue and the pointing finger.

—TOBA BETA

Whitmont writes:

> *The shadow is the door to our individuality. In so far as the shadow renders us our first view of the unconscious part of our personality, it represents the first stage toward meeting the Self. There is, in fact, no access to the unconscious and to our own reality but through the shadow.*[10]

When facing our shadow, we may experience any number of possible reactions. We can refuse to face it. We can notice it and try to eliminate it. We can refuse to accept any responsibility for it, and let it run us. Or we can, as Whitmont notes, "'suffer' it in a constructive manner, as a part of our personality which can lead us to a salutary humility and humanness and eventually to new insights and expanded life horizons."[11]

Refusal to face our shadow will lead to increased isolation and a projection of the world through our shadow's eyes. A vicious cycle of projections will then begin, shaping our attitude to others, which in turn creates the expected response and vicious cycle of "creating our own reality." But encounters with our shadow side can make the conscious personality feel shattered and overwhelmed. This is where humility serves us well.

Pride is considered one of the deadly sins, with good reason. If there are no more lessons to be learned, we begin to justify our behavior through acts of superiority or aloofness. In turn, this creates an opportunity for the universe to bring on valuable lessons of humility. Edward Bach suggested, "Pride is due, firstly, to lack of recognition of the smallness of the personality and its utter dependence on the Soul…. As Pride invariably refuses to bend with humility and resignation to the Will of the Great Creator, it commits actions contrary to that Will."[12] Alas, this vicious cycle continues its downward emotional spiral toward isolation, deceit, and conceit.

This pattern may begin early in life, especially if there has been lack of nurturance, or injury growing up. Wounded egos tend to act more confident than they really are, as a form of compensation.

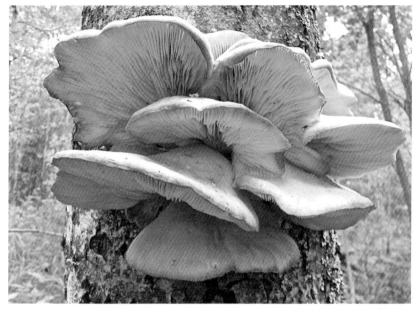

Older oyster mushroom

Essence description

Oyster mushroom essence is useful for issues involving humility and pride. It is the mushroom essence that allows us to see our true self. This is no easy step and involves recognition, connection, and acceptance of our shadow. Oyster mushroom essence helps open a variety of opportunities to reexamine our relationship with shadow.

The mushroom essence may help soften and soothe us emotionally, in difficult times of transition involving separation from loved ones, loss of career, divorce, and other painful moments on our earthly journey. It will not help us avoid the pain, but will soften the intensity.

Oyster mushroom essence helps us distinguish between the pretense of humility and the transformative nature of truly feeling its presence. The essence may be useful for inner work involving meditation, dream work, journaling, and other expressions of inner self-awareness.

The mycelium of pride has several branches. One of the largest is arrogance. Arrogant people create emotional walls to fend off hurt and criticism. Oyster mushroom essence may be useful in several ways. It may help spark the fire of discontent that accompanies attitudes of superiority and all-knowing intellectual egotism. This fire may begin to rage and burn up old perceptions of self and leave us with the ashes of destruction, if not handled with care. Without this catalyst, however, there would be no need to search for the quenching waters of emotion. Diving into the pool of self-awareness may be the result of attempting to cool down our fires of discontent.

Care must be used with oyster mushroom essence, as the elements of fire and water are powerful indeed. Manifestations of burning and drowning may appear in our reality as representations of this inner void and ensuing conflict with soul. Caution around fires and water is strongly recommended when using this essence.

Oyster mushroom essence may help address issues surrounding pride and arrogance by offering the opportunity for acceptance and gratefulness in our life. G. I. Gurdjieff noted that we have but two options in life. We can create the opportunity for small shocks of awareness, or the universe will provide us with larger shocks.[13]

Oyster mushroom essence helps pierce the armor of pride and arrogance, and set us on a more soulful path. It creates the mental and emotional atmosphere needed to bring awareness to our own attention, or lack thereof.

PREPARATION: This mushroom essence is produced from the wild fruiting body placed gills-down in a crystal bowl containing rainwater when the moon is in Leo (pride), or Scorpio (shadow). Leave it overnight. Remove the fruiting body with chopsticks and combine the rainwater one-to-one with brandy to make a mother essence.

CASE STUDY: Ted was a fifty-five-year-old man, married, with a stepson. He was the middle child in his family. He had previously consulted me for recurring winter bouts of bronchitis and pneumonia. His mother had recently died, but they had been estranged for over twenty years. Her will removed him from any inheritance, even though the money was insignificant. His arrogance was notable, from his overall demeanor to the manner in which he spoke of other people. He constantly berated their intelligence, belief systems, and lifestyles, as if he had exclusive insights into how a person lives. He was a committed atheist and proud of it. There was a significant issue of depression, and yet he felt superior to others. I suggested he take oyster mushroom essence for a lunar cycle and, surprisingly, he agreed.

He stopped taking it after four days, he told me later, as his experiences were too frightening and intense. He had a dream about drowning, and I asked him if he had ever experienced this trauma as a young boy. He did not recall any incident. I asked him to take only two drops daily and observe his reactions to people around him.

At the end of the cycle he returned to my office, a noticeably more humble individual. He had another dream of drowning, of falling through the ice, and seeing his reflection in the mirrorlike frozen surface. He said to me, "I know that religion is bogus, but if it gives comfort to people, there's nothing wrong with that." We agreed that this was a good beginning.

PSILOCYBE SPECIES

INDICATIONS: addiction, authority figures, consumerism, dancing, fear, denial

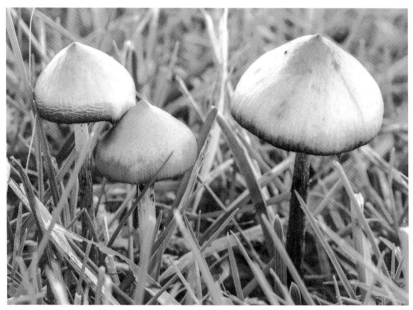

Liberty cap (*Psilocybe semilanceata* [Fries] P. Kummer) (courtesy of Caleb Brown)

Laws, like the spider's web, catch the fly and let the hawk go free.
—SPANISH PROVERB

If you don't have a plan, you become part of somebody else's plan.
—TERENCE MCKENNA

Dance is the hidden language of the soul of the body.
—MARTHA GRAHAM

According to Eric Dubay:

> *Libertus is a mushroom hero whose depiction can be found atop the U.S. Capitol Building, of all places. Libertus wears a liberty cap (or Phrygian cap) shaped like and named after the liberty cap mushroom. This is where we get the idea of a "thinking cap" because when you ingest the cap you are teleported into an introspective, wondrous experience. The Phrygian/liberty cap was worn by Masonic revolutionaries during the French and American revolutions as well as by Perseus, Mithra, Santa, Elves, and of course, Smurfs. It is worn as a "night cap," a double entendre which nowadays means having an alcoholic beverage before bed. The original idea of a night cap, however, was when Mithraic/Mystery school initiates would eat a large mushroom cap then lay in hot tubs and astrally project out of body.[14]*

It is ironic that people living in a democracy fear authority figures. Social media continues to capture video of police brutality, with little change to the political structure that ensures the rich and powerful continue to control people's lives. Martin W. Ball writes:

> *Western cultures' denigration of entheogens is related to the fear of the Shadow. That we live in a high state of denial and repression and fear is a major factor in our societies, from political policy to consumerism and advertising. We live in a deep state of fear and refusal to look honestly into the darkness of ourselves and seek to learn from what we find there. Cynically, this fear is widely manipulated in Western cultures, often to advantage of those in power. Fear keeps us obedient and passive to the powers that be. Do they have something to lose when people learn to free themselves from their fears and look honestly at reality?[15]*

Nearly forty years ago, I drove a Volkswagen beetle for one summer. I did not actually own it; it was a loaner from a friend. It had a bumper sticker, "Question Authority," which expressed the attitude of many fellow hippies in the early 1970s. I remember repeatedly being stopped and hassled by the police nearly every time I ventured onto the

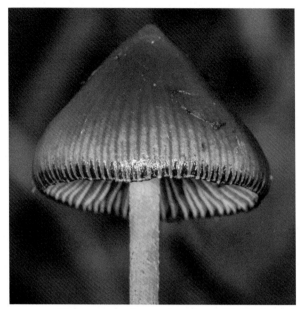

Liberty cap mushroom (courtesy of Caleb Brown)

highway. Reluctantly, I scraped off the sticker. Lesson learned, or so I thought. Fear and anxiety of authority figures is related to our own personal sense of power.

Essence description

Liberty cap mushroom essence does not, of course, contain any entheo-genic substance. But it does retain the energetic pattern associated with alleviating fear–associated issues surrounding authority figures. This essence is particularly liberating to individuals who suffer anxiety or resistance in their dealings with politicians, clergy, lawyers, judges, bankers, insurance agents, the constabulary, and others representing authority. It combines well with fly agaric mushroom essence for this specific issue.

Most individuals are simply doing their jobs, and are so fixated on doing it well, they are unaware of how they affect other people. It is not their issue. With maturity of soul, authority becomes an internal process that is owned and nurtured. There are exceptions, of course, and in some cases, abuse of power does take place.

Liberty cap mushroom essence helps us connect with our own sense of inner power and observe how others play their own role in the unfolding of human drama. In fact, taking liberty cap mushroom essence for a lunar cycle may allow us to positively attract individuals in positions of power. This will assist in helping break a long-standing pattern of fear, possibly related to past lives or early childhood interactions.

This mushroom essence is useful in helping individuals with shopping addictions. This is slightly different from drug and alcohol addictions, as may be imagined. Consumerism and buying things to fill an emotional void can range from minor to major addictive behavior. The phrase "You deserve it" has become an advertising mantra for companies pitching their wares. Plotkin writes:

> The most highly prized freedom is the right to shop. It's a world of commodities, not entities, and economic expansion is the primary measure of progress. Competition, taking, and hoarding are higher values than cooperation, sharing, and gifting. Profits are valued over people, money over meaning.[16]

Our educational, government, and corporate institutions support finance-based culture and are not interested in teaching people to live empowered lives.

One peculiar indication for this essence is the need to dance wherever there is music. The cure, of course, is dancing. Tarantism is related to overcoming melancholy by dancing, related to the behavior exhibited in sixteenth-century Italy by individuals bitten by a tarantula spider. Trance dancing can help us develop a relationship with soul. Everything in the universe dances: particles, amoebas, and cells all respond to the music of the universe.

PREPARATION: This fungal essence is produced from mature caps of liberty cap, with rainwater in a crystal singing bowl with the tone of middle C, during the full moon or lunar influence in Libra. Resonate the bowl as often as possible during the night.

NOTE: There are a wide range of entheogenic *Psilocybe*, *Panaeolus*, and *Stropharia* mushroom species, all with different constituents, temperaments, and personalities. There is much to explore in the wide range of individual gifts they offer. An entire book could be researched and written on various Psilocybe mushroom essences.

CASE STUDY: Melissa was a thirty-four-year-old single mother, recently separated, with two young children. She came to my clinic asking for help with right-side headaches. After a thorough review, I suggested there were indications of liver and gall bladder stress. She said her mother had her gall bladder removed at age forty-five. But there was something else. She finally broke down in tears and revealed that her husband had hired a very expensive lawyer and was harassing her about child support and custody. She was barely making ends meet, and it seemed to her the whole legal system was her enemy. I suggested she take liberty cap mushroom essence for a lunar cycle, and also asked her to keep a dream journal.

The shift in energy she experienced was profound. Within three days she met, by chance, an old high school friend, and through a chain of events was then introduced to her lawyer husband. Within two weeks, he, as her lawyer, had demanded a meeting with the husband's lawyer, and the tide of the entire proceeding shifted in her favor. Her headaches stopped.

One day, she was listening to the radio, and a favorite song began to play; she found herself dancing around the kitchen in joyful exuberance. She felt alive again.

FLY AGARIC

(Amanita muscaria)

INDICATIONS: expansion, contraction, sexual abuse, rejection, self-expression, religion, creativity, pain, insecurity, Dupuytren's contracture, arthritis, scleroderma

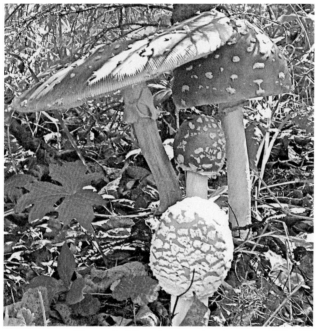

Fly agaric (*Amanita muscaria* var. guessowii Veselý)

The object of therapeutic treatment is to return imagination to the things that have become only physical.
—ROBERT SARDELLO

The improver of natural knowledge absolutely refuses to acknowledge authority, as such. For him, skepticism is the highest of duties; blind faith the one unpardonable sin.
—THOMAS HENRY HUXLEY

Expansion and contraction are states of being that manifest on physical, mental, emotional, spiritual, and soul-centered planes. The body and brain respond to signals of loosening and tightening based on their physical and mental needs and messages sent to various organ systems.

Research has found social pain, rejection, grieving, and the end of affairs or relationships can trigger these types of reactions. The dorsal anterior cingulate part of the brain is associated with the sensation of pain. Work by James A. Coan at the University of Virginia found that when the patients' hands were held by their loved ones, their perception of pain lessened, as did the neural response in the dorsal anterior cingulate. In troubled relationships, this protection did not occur.[17] Holding and viewing a photograph of a significant other also reduced experimentally induced pain.[18]

Social rejection is interpreted by the brain like a threat of physical harm, suggesting that episodes of rejection can be as damaging and debilitating as episodes of physical pain.

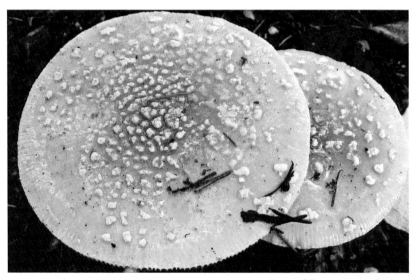

Caps of fly agaric mushroom

Essence description

Fly agaric mushroom essence is related to natural phases of expansion and contraction. The mushroom essence is particularly useful when early childhood trauma is related to abuse by authority figures. This could be of a physical, mental, or emotional nature and inflicted by parents, relatives, teachers, ministers, priests, group leaders—basically, any older adult representing authority and protection. There may be associated difficulty with self-expression and fear of criticism by others. The feelings of insecurity and lack of safety as well as mistrust imprint upon the immature psyche and may fuel lifelong dysfunction.

Physical and sexual abuse are two obvious situations, but abuse can be more subtle when associated with various mental and emotional planes. An unconscious negative remark from a schoolteacher, for example, may leave the scar of limitations on the young mind. An unkind, ill-thought-out aside from a parent may leave a lasting impression and limit our potential. One example is the remark "You're so stupid." This may evolve and revolve in the young impressionable mind, leading to difficulty with studies or affecting feelings of self-worth.

Fly agaric mushroom essence may be useful for individuals who resent or retain negative emotions associated with politicians, lawyers, bankers, police, and financially successful members of society. It combines well with liberty cap for this particular issue. A repeating mantra in the mind that life is unfair, or resentment over other people's success, can undermine our ability to move forward and create our own success.

On a mental level, the mushroom essence may help increase expansion or contraction of thought patterns. Expansion is necessary for imagination and creativity. Contraction is related to concrete action or editing thoughts and words associated with writing.

On an emotional level, fly agaric essence helps us to become more generous and expansive in thought and deed. Giving of ourselves is a special gift. Repeated patterns associated with early childhood trauma may reinforce the need to be guarded and protect ourselves. This can lead to hardening of attitudes and result in contraction, constriction, and even greater need for control.

Dupuytren's contracture, for example, is a tightening of tendons and ligaments of the hands. There is hardening of attitude as well as pointing of the finger, associated with criticism and inflexibility. Various muscular and joint conditions such as arthritis, rheumatoid arthritis, and scleroderma may be helped with fly agaric mushroom essence.

Spiritually, fly agaric mushroom essence assists us in overcoming early religious training that led to rebellion or resistance to our own spiritual path. It is not a coincidence that early Christian cults were awash in fly agaric consumption. Three books of note for those who would like to explore this relationship are Clark Heinrich's *Magic Mushrooms in Religion and Alchemy,* John A. Rush's *The Mushroom in Christian Art,* and J. R. Irvin and Jack Herer's *The Holy Mushroom.*[19]

On the spiritual plane, there is an ebb and flow that feels like expansion and contraction. In the former state, it feels like life is flowing and each new adventure is positive and fulfilling. This is the result of listening to our intuition. *Intuition* comes from the Latin *intueri,* meaning "to examine," but has come to be associated with an inner voice or a shortcut to reason.

This may be followed by contraction of self, resulting in depression, anger or numbness, and the inability to accept difficult situations. This is a state of ego, based on the need to control ourselves and those around us, moving even farther away from connection with soul.

Fly agaric mushroom essence may ease the tremor of Parkinson's disease, in a manner similar to the highly potentiated homeopathic preparations. Note that this condition is an over-firing of neurons, while Alzheimer's disease is associated with a lack of neural connection. For senile dementia, and loss of both short- and long-term memory, think of comb tooth mushroom essence.

PREPARATION: This mushroom essence is prepared by inverting the mature caps and filling them with rainwater. This is left overnight during a full moon, and then the water is removed with a dropper and stabilized with equal parts of brandy.

CASE STUDY: Randy was seventy-four years old, a widower, and formerly a cement worker. He came to my clinic for help with severe osteoarthritis in both knees. He was taking six to eight Tylenol daily, and liver tests were indicating hepatotoxicity and tissue destruction. He was looking for any alternative. I suggested nettle leaf, which gave him the same level of pain relief with half doses of Tylenol, and milk thistle for liver detoxification and regeneration. A month later he began

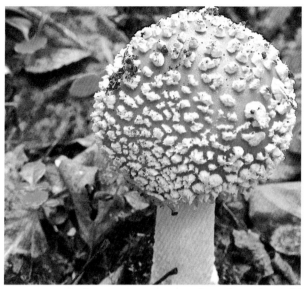

Immature fly agaric just emerging from the underworld

to take Solomon's seal rhizome tincture to begin the regeneration of synovial fluid and cartilage tissue.

After three months there was significant improvement, but Randy was still suffering immense emotional contraction. He admitted to me that since the death of his wife three years earlier, life was not the same. He felt numb, angry, and depressed, and believed life was being unfair. I recommended he take fly agaric mushroom essence for a lunar cycle.

His next visit showed vast improvement in his emotional and mental health. He talked about a trip to Europe to visit his ancestors' home village. He felt it was time to do something "concrete" with his life. I had to laugh.

FAIRY RING

(Marasmius oreades)

INDICATIONS: birth, fertility, inner child, menstruation, circadian rhythm, melatonin, pregnancy, labor

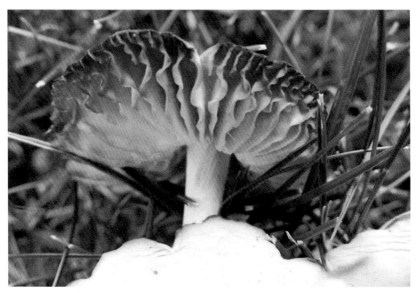

Fairy ring (*Marasmius oreades* [Bolton] Fries)

It is never too late to have a happy childhood.

—OLD SAYING

Where round the bed, whence Achelous springs,
That watery Fairies dance in mazy things.

—HOMER, ILIAD 24

He who knows the masculine but keeps to the
feminine will be in the whole world's channel.

—TAOIST SAYING

All of nature, including human beings, is subject to seasonal, lunar, and circadian rhythms. The lunar cycle has been poorly explored and yet has important influence on human behavior and physiology. Fertility, menstruation, and birth rates in women are influenced by phases of the moon. Lunacy, as a condition of mental health, has been correlated with the full moon. Mushrooms are no different. It has been found that daily variations in melatonin and corticosterone in birds disappear during full moon days.[20] Nor Hall (1980) writes:

We know what the ebb and flow of psychic energy (the energy of psyche or soul) feels like. A rhythm of constant change, the waxing and waning of creativity, of love of life, of the ability to be with people, of our alertness and sexuality and health—these periodic changes of mood and being, characterize the feminine principle. It is moist, cool, receptive, and then passionate and inflaming like fire. It is alternately full and available—shedding a steady radiant light—and dark and distant, untouchable.[21]

Humans respond to the lunar tides of emotion. Males have cycles as well, but these are twenty-two days in length, and relate to weight loss and changes in the albumen levels in urine. Hall continues:

Watching the moon in the course of its monthly growth and diminishing in a way of reminding ourselves that the periodic need to be in-full-view and the opposite periodic need to be alone or withdrawn are not only natural but essential to the feminine. I am taking care to say "the feminine" here rather than "female" or "womanly" to stress its roving home. Femininity is a mode of being human that can be lived out (and betrayed or suppressed) by both men and women.[22]

Difficulties associated with irregular periods, fertility issues, pregnancy, or labor may be helped with fairy ring mushroom essence.

Fairy rings have long been associated with the full moon, dancing in circles, and other mythology. An interesting association of protection is noted inside the circle and outside. Another signature is the ability of the fruiting body to spring back to life with a new rain. The dehydrated and withered body becomes plump and full, ready to complete its reproductive task.

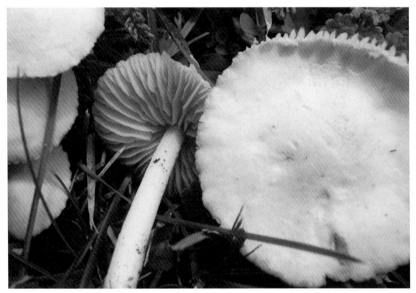

Fairy ring mushrooms

Essence description

Fairy ring mushroom essence relates to our connection with our inner child. Early childhood wounds, imagined or real, can influence our response and attitudes throughout life. Fairy ring mushroom essence helps create balance between the masculine and feminine in everyone. Connecting with our wounded inner child, and assuring them they are now protected, helps adults begin to appreciate the small joys and wonders of life once again. The essence helps reestablish childlike trust and freedom in the older adult. It helps us learn to play again.

The essence helps us feel protected and be a protector of our loved ones. It is useful for mother and child during pregnancy, whenever external influences are negative in nature.

Imagine the sensation of release dancing with the little ones around a fairy ring under a full moon. If you cannot conjure up this inner vision without a smile, this may be your mushroom essence. Fairy ring combines well with liberty cap for those individuals who would like to dance but are fearful of doing so in a public setting. Try it!

PREPARATION: The mushroom essence is prepared with fruiting caps in a crystal bowl filled with rainwater, centered inside a fairy ring on a full moon night. Ideally, this would be with the moon in the signs of Cancer or Pisces.

CASE STUDY: Linda was twenty-four years old, married, with fertility problems. She was suffering irregular menstrual cycles, had experienced two miscarriages in two years, and felt dejected, defeated, and upset. She was also deeply religious. I asked her if she believed in angels, to which she nodded affirmatively. I then asked if she believed in fairies. She looked startled, looked at her husband, and softly said, "I guess so." I invited her to try fairy ring mushroom essence for one lunar cycle, keep a dream journal, and then come back to see me.

Her next visit was most interesting. About ten days into taking the essence, she told me, she had a dream in which she saw herself as a six- or seven-year-old, watching her own mother suffer a miscarriage, complete with excessive blood all over the bathroom floor. The memory startled and woke her, accompanied by a shivering sweat. A week later this same young girl appeared in her dream, telling her schoolyard friends that she was never going to get pregnant. Again, she awoke in panicked mode. I invited her to connect with her younger inner child when the opportunity presented itself again. Sixteen months later, she delivered a healthy baby girl.

AGARICUS SPECIES

INDICATIONS: alienation, attention, survival, stress, awareness, zest, hyperactivity, nature-deficit disorder, urban-rural disconnect, biomedicine, veterinary medicine, Ritalin

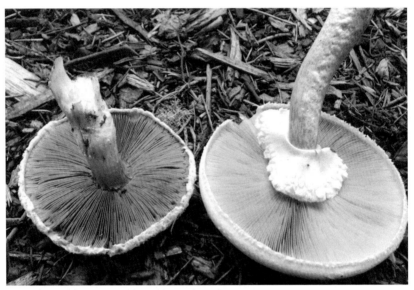

Agaricus campestris (L.) and *A. sylvicola* (Vittadini) Peck: the tamed and the wild

"Men have forgotten this truth," said the fox. "But you must not forget it. You become responsible, forever, for what you have tamed."

—ANTOINE DE SAINT-EXUPÉRY

Teaching children about the natural world should be treated as one of the most important events in their lives.

—THOMAS BERRY

I grew up in a city. I played baseball on an asphalt playground near my elementary school. It was only after I had completed my Bachelor of Science degree and moved to a rural hippie community in the early 1970s that I began to appreciate my own lack of connection with nature. I built a log home, learned to garden and wild-craft, raised rabbits, goats, and chickens, picked mushrooms, and lived without electricity or running water for a few years. It was an important passage, helping me come of age.

Louv writes, "Nature-deficit disorder describes the human costs of alienation from nature, among them: diminished use of the senses, attention difficulties, and higher rates of physical and emotional illnesses."[23] One of the great shifts for humankind was our transition from hunter-gatherer to an agricultural society. This shift has been both a blessing and a curse. On the plus side, the increased availability of food led to massive cultural and technological growth. Day-to-day survival was no longer a constant concern in most of the developed world. But something was lost. People became increasingly separated from, and in many cases, alienated from nature. Children, it is said, can name up to fifty corporate logos, and yet would be hard-pressed to name three mushrooms on the school playground—or even know how to identify a mushroom.

The last two generations of children educated in our public school system have lost touch with their wild side. They seek enjoyment from controlling a joystick or a computer game that is artificial in its rewards. In turn, this has led vast numbers of people to consider themselves separate from nature and to condone the exploitation and destruction of wilderness as the price to pay for civilization and the "good life."

In some quarters, the idea that nature has to be tamed is still prevalent, that somehow muscle and brawn are needed to brave this unpredictable wild world. And yet very few males with machismo could spend a single night in the woods by themselves. Our connection with nature is an important antidote to fear. Becoming nature-smart and self-aware helps us separate imagined fear and anxiety from real physical danger.

Modern biomedicine is slowly recognizing that many of today's modern illnesses are stress-related and fear-based. But alas, many medical doctors are a leading cause of disease. This is largely due to a diminished approach of one-on-one connection and caring experience necessary to instill an optimal sense of empowerment in their patients. Doctors are not heroes, and patients do not have to be rescued.

Agaricus was the first mushroom domesticated for human consumption. The common button mushroom is found in every supermarket in

North America, both loved and loathed. Its wild relatives are highly prized by mycophiles, who relish the more intense, robust flavor. The analogy could not be more obvious.

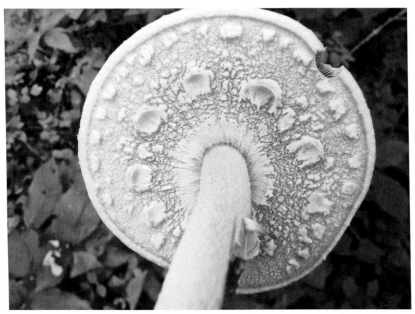

Agaricus campestris

Essence description

Agaricus mushroom essence helps restore balance and encourages an appreciation of nature. It can help restore a sense of calm in domesticated animals, both in the barnyard and for companion animals in an urban home.

Agaricus mushroom essence helps us accept and embrace our wild side, in a respectful manner that appreciates the demands of modern society. It helps create the mental capacity necessary to observe and feel equally at home in the city or the forest. Agaricus combines well with artist's conk for issues involving levels of comfort in nature.

The combination of field and forest Agaricus mushroom essences relates to the concept of domestication, taming, and the compulsive need to control ourselves and nature. It is important to note that tameness may relate to domestication, or to the need to soften or tone down.

It may also relate to deprivation of courage, zest, or excitement, resulting in disinterest in life and automatically going through the basic motions of living.

Agaricus mushroom essence helps us break our addiction to television. A client may well rationalize and reject our opinions, like any addict deprived of their fix. Computer games fall into the same category. There is good reason to examine this issue. Plotkin writes, "Television ranks high among the common addictions in our society, along with the other 'screen' obsessions: the internet, PalmPilots, and videos."[24] I would add smart phones to this list. Berendt notes that TV people become onlookers, not participants. It is a modern attitude to remain at a distance, uninvolved, and alienated.[25] This attitude is in the interest of the powers that be. Viewers become chained or cabled down to indifference and desensitization. These particular addicts will come up with any number of excuses to continue their removal from intimate, soulful connection. Agaricus mushroom essence may help us break this addiction, and it combines well with turkey tail mushroom essence.

Agaricus mushroom essence may help initiate regeneration of our deeper levels of awareness and consciousness. It may invigorate the primal forces that give meaning to survival instincts, and instill wildness and wilderness back into the human psyche.

Agaricus mushroom essence may be helpful in weaning "hyperactive" children from Ritalin and related medications, under the supervision of a health practitioner. Combine with algae maze mushroom essence for enhanced benefit.

PREPARATION: This mushroom essence is produced using field and forest Agaricus species under moonlight. Wild and tame fruiting bodies are placed in one crystal bowl filled with rainwater for one night, under the influence of Taurus or Sagittarius. If you cannot find field mushrooms, you may substitute organic cremini button mushrooms. Slice these tame Agaricus members thinly with a ceramic knife and place them on top of rainwater as above.

The energetics of commercially produced mushrooms will vary widely due to the multitude of personalities involved in growing, harvesting, shipping, and touching them in a store. The same is true of commercial shiitake and Cordyceps mushrooms. It is interesting to note that shiitake, imported initially from Japan and widely cultivated in North America, has "escaped" into the forests of North and South Carolina. Yeah!

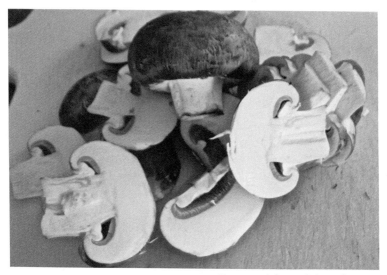

Commercial cremini mushrooms

CASE STUDY: Sean was a thirty-seven-year-old single graphic designer working in animation. He came to my clinic for help with carpal tunnel syndrome. He was left-handed, and the pain and inflammation was much worse in that wrist. Surgery was suggested by his family physician. I suggested he try preformed vitamin B6, pyridoxal 5′-phosphate, for one month and see if there was any improvement. He returned in less than a month with significant improvement and was very pleased he could avoid surgery.

He asked me if I had any suggestions for help with his fear of the outdoors. He lived downtown on the twenty-sixth floor of a high-rise. His successful animation company was in the same building on the eighth floor, so he rarely left the building except for shopping and food. I asked him when he had last experienced an outdoor adventure, and he replied that it was about three years before, when he went on a skiing trip to the mountains. I suggested that he may be suffering nature-deficit disorder, and he laughed and asked, "Is that a clinical diagnosis"? I suggested Agaricus mushroom essence might help him reconnect with nature and his wild side. He was unsure what I meant, but he was willing to try it, as I had helped him with his painful wrist. I asked him to take the mushroom essence once daily each evening, and then go for an hour's walk on the nearby river valley trails.

One month later he returned to my office. His previously clean-shaven face was fuzzy with a sprouting beard, and he was wearing blue jeans and a flannel shirt. I asked him about his experience with the mushroom essence. He'd had a nightmare one night, he said, in which he was about ten years old and camping with his parents and siblings. They awoke to the sounds of two mature black bears rummaging through their food containers. He remembered never being so terrified in his life. I suggested that this was great progress and that he continue his daily hour-long walks and take another lunar cycle of Agaricus mushroom essence. He agreed. We saw each other for the next half year and mainly worked with various flower and mushroom essences.

Eight months later he came to my office and introduced me to his girlfriend, a local botanist and photographer he met on one of his pre-scribed walks. He had sold his multimillion-dollar shares in the animation company and was presently in a venture to build a neighborhood brewpub. I congratulated him and wished both of them a happy life. As he was leaving the office I mentioned that the yeast used in making beer was part of the kingdom Fungi. "Mushrooms are addictive," I said. We all laughed.

VELVET FOOT
(Flammulina populicola)

INDICATIONS: discomfort, materialism, nakedness, responsibility, skin, psoriasis, eczema, discontent

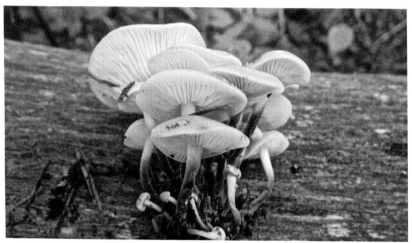

Velvet foot (*Flammulina populicola* Redhead & R. H. Petersen)

Restlessness is discontent and discontent is the first necessity of progress. Show me a thoroughly satisfied man and I will show you a failure.
—THOMAS A. EDISON

Healthy discontent is the prelude to progress.
—MAHATMA GANDHI

You can be still and still moving. Content even in your discontent.
—RAM DASS

Years may wrinkle the skin, but to give up enthusiasm wrinkles the soul.
—SAMUEL ULLMAN

Velvet Foot is a close relative of the cultivated medicinal mushroom enoki (*F. velutipes*). An epidemiological study in Japan found the lowest rates of all forms of cancer were centered on a city where enoki are produced.

Western culture has confused contentment with the accumulation of wealth. Happiness is something we cultivate, day by day. We sow the seeds of promise and carefully tend our garden (soul). We ensure the water of emotion is plentiful, and the heat and passion of the sun will take care of the rest. And all the while, the underground mycelial mats of soul connection help to nurture and protect.

Essence description

Velvet foot mushroom essence is related to the qualities of contentment. This quality of being is a source of much confusion in our modern materialistic world. Contentment has little to do with external trappings of wealth, prestige, or privilege. It has very little to do with inflated ego or learning how to play out societal roles.

Velvet foot essence helps us to connect and discern within the conflicts of conscience that help develop personal and moral responsibility. There is often confusion between our clothing (pseudo-ego) and our skin, resulting in ethical dilemmas. It may appear somewhat easy to wrap ourselves in the persona of expectations provided by society. And on the other hand, it is also somewhat easy to refuse to play any assigned roles that we associate with success.

The inner peace of soul connection is felt when we do our best, even in difficult situations. It is the positive consequence that results when we walk our talk.

Velvet foot helps us uncover dreams of clothing, such as being unable to take off clothing, or being overdressed, or wearing heavy uniforms. Alternatively, the dreams may find us exposed and naked at a party, or walking around in a transparent gown.

Persona and shadow are opposites. Identifying too much with either extreme can lead to false contentment associated with the social role in life, or a degree of discontent leading to compulsive or more primitive behavior. Neither is very useful for soul growth.

Our skin is our boundary, our connection with the external world and our sense of self. Skin conditions can manifest along with distortions of this pattern, including dermatitis, eczema, psoriasis, and granuloma. The essence may be dropped into ointments or salves to help with these issues. In some cases it combines well with snake liverwort.

PREPARATION: Velvet foot mushroom essence is prepared overnight in ice cold rainwater in a crystal bowl during a new moon in Libra or Capricorn.

CASE STUDY: Nancy was forty-two years old, married, with two teenagers, working part-time as a medical receptionist. She came to my clinic for help with chronic psoriasis. It was particularly thickened on her elbows, knees, scalp, and back of the neck. She had used cortisone creams for years, but the skin in these areas was getting very thin. Herbal and dietary approaches helped somewhat but the problem was persistent. After four months of limited success, I decided to dig a little deeper. I noted that she always over-dressed, obviously covering up the unsightly plaques. I suggested a lunar cycle of velvet foot mushroom essence. She liked the name, so she agreed. About a week later she phoned and was very distraught. Her psoriasis had flared up and was inflamed. I asked her if she had experienced any unusual dreams. She responded flippantly, "Oh, well, the usual one where I'm naked at a party." I suggested she come to see me for an appointment.

I asked if she was contented with life. She responded that she was very content, having enough money, family, and friends, in that order. I asked about her career, and she said it was "just a job." I asked her if she had any passions or hobbies she enjoyed in her spare time. She confided to me that she had always wanted to write poetry. I suggested she take a little time each day to pursue this no-longer-secret love. Over the next eight months her psoriasis became negligible, sometimes flaring with dietary indiscretions. Two years later she published a book of poetry called *Skin Deep*. She gave me a signed copy.

WRINKLED PEACH

(Rhodotus palmatus)

INDICATIONS: relationships, well-being, freedom, self-love, unconditionality, resistance, catalyst

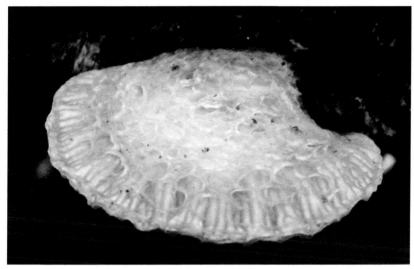

Wrinkled peach (*Rhodotus palmatus* [Bulliard] Maire)

*I demand unconditional love and complete
freedom. That is why I am terrible.*
—TOMAŽ ŠALAMUN

*When you focus on someone's disability you'll overlook their abilities,
beauty, and uniqueness. Once you learn to accept and love them for
who they are, you subconsciously learn to love yourself unconditionally.*
—YVONNE PIERRE

*Accept the children the way we accept trees—with gratitude, because
they are a blessing—but do not have expectations or desires.
You don't expect trees to change, you love them as they are.*
—ISABEL ALLENDE

Our happiness does not depend on the opinions or judgment of others. Love, for example, is a feeling and can thus be unconditional. Relationships are working partnerships and require boundaries, limits, and conditions in order to run smoothly. For some individuals, love is enough and is unconditional. For others, experiencing love and working on creating a healthy relationship takes work and the healthy exchange of ideas, negotiations, and setting boundaries.

Plotkin writes, "Egocentric romance is so common and compelling in the initiation-deprived Western world because the uninitiated ego approaches romance from the perspective of its own experience, which is one of deficiency and incompleteness."[26] Unconditionality is selfish in that our own well-being is the most important decision. It increases our sense of freedom and does not limit choices. In fact, we can be in a state of unconditionality and yet wish for things to change. We can accept the moment as it presents itself and still have the free will and the ability to react and choose differently. This changes the outcome. It allows us to increase scope and create the inner experience we crave despite our external world. Plotkin continues,

> Through its extreme currents and emotions, romance destabilizes the ego and opens a door to soul. Romance can be engaged soulfully and consciously, or it can be engaged egocentrically. When approached egocentrically, we unknowingly project aspects of our selves and our parents onto our beloved and thus have a limited understanding of the real person with whom we are partnered…. We fervently believe an intimate engagement with a lover is the thing that will save us, complete us, or make our world right.[27]

Essence description

Wrinkled peach mushroom essence is related to the quality of unconditionality. This concept is widely misunderstood. This confusion arises from focusing on what we are doing, and not on how we are being. That is, unconditional love arises from a state of mind. It is a powerful tool, because we cannot always control situations, but we can always change our mind. This is the great lesson shared by my father.

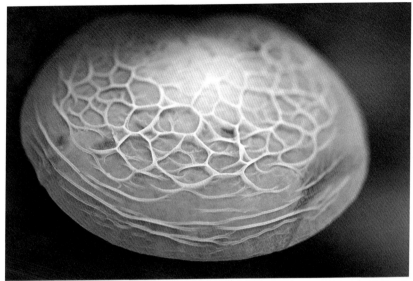

Wrinkled peach (courtesy of Alan McClelland)

"You have two choices in life—change your situation or change your mind," he often said.

It often comes down to resisting or allowing. Allowing feels good, light, and refreshing; resistance is heavy, tense, and futile. Wrinkled peach mushroom essence helps us commit to unconditionality in life. When this shift occurs, we become empowered from the inside out.

Wrinkled peach mushroom essence is valuable for individuals or two or more people in a relationship to take at the same time. Western society's romance involves a belief that we are each half people, and that by finding our other half, we are made whole. This romantic adolescent notion is reinforced in modern movies and music.

This mushroom essence is of great value to the psychologist or counselor working with couples who are working through difficulties. Issues involving affairs, abuse, and addictions put considerable strain on trust in relationships, including marriage.

Wrinkled peach can be used as a catalyst to bring issues to the surface and allow them to boil over, rather than continue to simmer endlessly. Care must be exercised, as "popping the cork" can be intense and dramatic. Like other mushroom essences, the issues of wrinkled peach relate to self-love. It is simply not possible to love another if it is lacking in ourselves. However, love is the door that opens us to soul connection.

PREPARATION: Wrinkled peach mushroom essence is created in a rain-water-filled crystal bowl, under lunar influence of Libra for one night whenever it is found.

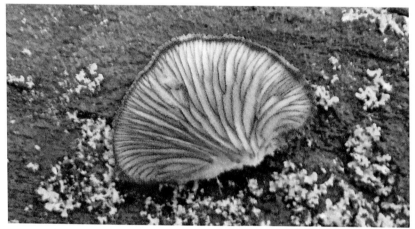

Gill side of a wrinkled peach

CASE STUDY: Amy was a twenty-five-year-old single flight attendant. She came to see me as she was having trouble with her boyfriend of seven years. She said she loved him, but felt that he was not "in love" with her. I asked her what that looked like. She confided that she worked very hard to please and make him happy, and yet he did not do the same. I suggested she experience a lunar cycle of wrinkled peach mushroom essence and she agreed.

She came to see me ten days later, very upset and angry. She said, "I blame you for breaking up my perfect relationship." I replied, "Don't you mean *your* perfect relationship?" She froze, and her entire body began to shudder as if in the first stages of a seizure. This soon abated, and was quickly followed by deep sobbing and tears that went on for a few minutes. I asked her if she loved him, to which she nodded. I asked her if she loved herself, and she did not answer.

I suggested that she needed to share this information with him and recognize love is a feeling and can be unconditional. I suggested it was possible that her trying so hard to make things work was causing him to feel pressured. I suggested she take one more lunar cycle of wrinkled peach mushroom essence.

Two months later, she came to see me and told me their relationship was over. I asked her how she felt. "Relieved," she replied. "I thought if I did everything right he would learn to love me."

Three months later, she met a young man whom she married two years later.

LOBSTER

(Hypomyces lactifluorum)

INDICATIONS: self-fulfilling prophecy, delusions, invisibility, zombies, vulnerability, occult, premature birth, exhaustion, astral travel

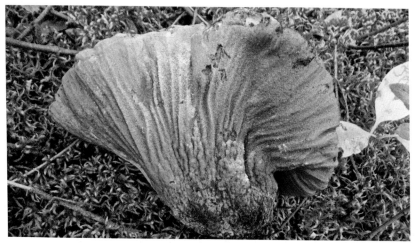

The lobster (*Hypomyces lactifluorum* [Schweinitz] Tulasne & C. Tulasne)

Europe's the mayonnaise, but America supplies the good old lobster.
—D. H. LAWRENCE

It's almost as if we each have a vampire inside us. Controlling that beast, that dark side, is what fascinates me.
—SHERYL LEE

I happen to like vampires more than zombies.
—MARTIN SCORSESE

Hypomyces lactifluorum is a fungus that is opportunistically parasitic on members of *Russula* and *Lactarius* genera. In the former, pictured above, the mushroom turns an edible, but less desirable, white *Russula brevipes* into a bright, florescent orange and highly prized edible mushroom.

It changes a gilled mushroom into something different. That is, a parasitic mushroom attacks another mushroom and creates something completely different.

Essence description

Lobster mushroom essence is useful for individuals born prematurely and who exhibit a weak astral body or etheric sheath (energy pattern) around them. That is, they have been brought onto the earthly plane before having any opportunity to develop their own strong sense of protection, and are thus more vulnerable to psychic impressions.

Early in life, these individuals may have invisible friends or talk to various plants and animals in a natural manner. They may, later in life, develop a fascination with vampires, zombies, and other symbolic manifestations of immortality. They may be drawn to the occult and delve into astrology, tarot, the I Ching, and other forms of divination. In fact, this mushroom essence is strongly associated with hexagram 24 in the I Ching system.

Modern society is full of zombies. We are told that free will is not possible and that we are really just zombies. We have forgotten how to think and feel, and of course, the zombies keep reminding us that we should not feel too much or think too deeply. Ignore the zombies.

Lobster mushroom essence helps strengthen our energetic field of protection. Although some individuals prefer to keep the veil between the worlds more accessible, this constant leakage of energy can, on many levels, become exhausting and debilitating. Physical and mental lethargy are commonplace. These individuals can become victims of their own delusions. And if, by chance, one of their "premonitions" comes to pass, the reality of self-fulfilling prophecy comes into being. This is not so much a result of the law of attraction, or negative attracting negative, as it is based on self-actualized fear.

Lobster mushroom essence acts as a psychic guard, promoting a feeling of safety and relaxation. Only then can we begin to investigate our own shadow, which, when encountered, feels like death to the ego.

Robert Bly said our first twenty years are spent stuffing 90 percent of our wholeness into "the long bag we drag behind us."[28] And then we spend the rest of our lives attempting to retrieve our true self. It is acknowledging these negative shadow pieces, and their conscious integration, that leads us to soul connection.

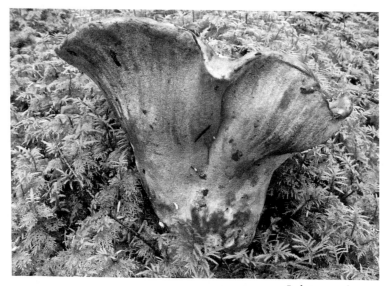

Lobster mushroom

PREPARATION: Lobster mushroom essence is best prepared by filling the concave open mushroom with rainwater anytime during the waxing period of the moon in lunar water signs, including Cancer. Brush out vegetative debris before filling it with water, and leave it overnight. This water is carefully drawn off the next morning and combined with equal parts of brandy.

CASE STUDY: Jodi was a thirty-three-year-old single government employee. She was born prematurely and adopted at a young age. Early in life she developed a fascination for the occult and psychic phenomenon. She came to see me suffering longtime fatigue. She did not exhibit the joint pain, tender chest points, and other symptoms of chronic fatigue syndrome, but she was constantly exhausted and suffered insomnia. She did not remember her dreams. I suggested she take lobster and bird's nest mushroom essences for a lunar cycle.

She returned, looking more refreshed and lively, her face no longer white and pale. She found the mushroom essence had helped her sleep, and her dreams were somewhat different. I asked her in what way. She said it was hard to explain but that she no longer felt exhausted from defending, protecting, and hiding in her dreams. One night, she found herself astral traveling over a city she had always wished to visit. She saw the name of a café on the corner of a street, complete with street sign. I invited her to consider traveling there one day.

Eight months later she did. She came to tell me what happened. She entered the café and immediately her body began to feel all tingly. She sat down and immediately met the eyes of the man sitting at the next table. He looked so familiar. They married six months later.

EARTH STAR

(Geastrum triplex)

INDICATIONS: addiction, cosmic connection, materialism, impulsiveness, optimism, extroversion, escapism, Jekyll-and-Hyde

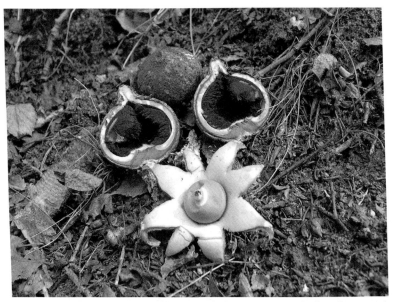

Earth star (*Geastrum triplex* Junghuhn) (courtesy of John Thompson)

There is a crack, a crack in everything. That's how the light gets in.
—LEONARD COHEN

The object of life is not to be on the side of the majority, but to escape finding oneself in the ranks of the insane.
—MARCUS AURELIUS

Earth Star mushrooms have either seven or eight points. Eight is the number of stability and earthiness, while seven is a combination of three, representing spirituality, and four, representing earthiness and symbols such as the cross, box, or square. Star shapes are wide open and suggest cosmic connection. Brown is the color of impermanence and outer worldliness, including death and rebirth.

Alcohol, marijuana, nicotine, heroin, cocaine, and addictive pharmaceutical drugs all give earth stars the escape they desperately desire. These individuals then attach themselves to people with similar addictions to feel a false sense of "friendship." Many have tried Alcoholics Anonymous (AA) or twelve-step-based treatment programs with limited success. This is not surprising. As Lance Dodes notes in *The Sober Truth,* "Every year, our state and federal governments spend over $15 billion on substance-abuse treatment for addicts, the vast majority of which are based on a twelve-step program. There is only one problem: these programs almost always fail."[1]

Other addictions follow similar patterns. Western society is increasingly materialistic, synthetic, technological, ethnocentric, and geocentric. It is difficult to fit into this paradigm without losing contact with soul. And thus, increasingly large numbers of people seek to numb themselves from their loss of connection with nature, the natural web of life, and their souls.

Essence description

Earth star mushroom essence may be helpful for the seemingly optimistic, extroverted, and playful individual. These individuals are constantly seeking new experiences and may suffer at times from impatience or impulsive behavior. Earth star people will do whatever is needed to maintain their freedom and happiness and avoid pain at all costs. When looking for answers outside themselves, they are generally spirit-seeking, but are not concerned or aware of soul-connection.

Earth star individuals care more about having a good time than seeking power, but they can become overly materialistic in the accumulation of fancy cars, homes, partners, and clothes. There is a distinct and hidden dark side to this disconnection from soul. Always the life of the party, they have a great deal of inner torment that is only sedated or relieved by an attraction to addictions. This may be especially true if a previous traumatic life event has occurred and the grief has been repressed. Loss of a loved one, for example, can lead earth star individuals to subconsciously desire to join with them on the next plane.

Extreme care must be used when taking this mushroom essence. It may act as a catalyst, bringing to awareness a deeply buried trauma.

Addictive personalities can easily slide between false persona and a truly Jekyll-and-Hyde demeanor. The largest lies they tell are to themselves. The original story, by Robert Louis Stevenson, is widely misunderstood. Jekyll really does want the freedom to be Hyde. Jekyll is a deeply disturbed and repressed man who does not want to suffer consequences, and is aware of what happens at night.

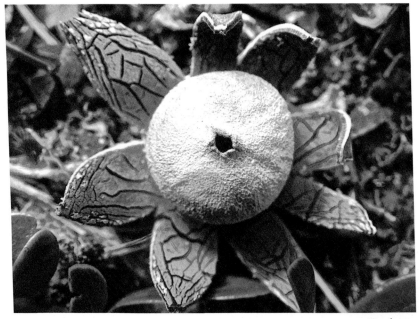

Earth star

PREPARATION: This mushroom essence is best taken throughout the day as needed, usually in doses of seven or eight drops at a time. The essence is prepared by placing both seven- and eight-pointed earth stars on top of rainwater in a crystal bowl.

Ideally this remedy is prepared at the new moon in Sagittarius. For alcohol addiction, you can remove the brandy by putting the drops in a cup of boiled water. The brandy will evaporate and can then be used. This is true of all the mushroom essences.

CASE STUDY: Gordon was a forty-five-year-old divorced stock market trader. He came to my office looking for help with addiction. He had struggled with substance abuse for over twenty years, starting with alcohol and marijuana, and progressing to cocaine and heroin use. He was presently limiting himself to alcohol (beer), marijuana, and cigarettes, one pack per day. He had been through two bouts of rehab, the latest following a DUI that resulted in him losing his driver's license for six months. I asked him if he could remember any traumatic event that preceded his addictive path, and he could not. I recommended he take earth star mushroom essence throughout the day and before bedtime for a lunar cycle. I also asked him to cut down by one cigarette a day until he was down to six. He agreed to try.

One month later he appeared in my office and had a different aura about him. He seemed more relaxed and comfortable. He was down to six cigarettes a day, and I congratulated him on that. He said he was no longer drinking alcohol, and I joked, "Except for the brandy in your remedy." He laughed and asked what we do next. "Did you have any dreams?" I asked. He could not remember any, but mentioned that one night he did have a night-time vision of his long-deceased friend from business school. I pursued this track, and he revealed his best friend, Jack, had died in a traffic accident when only twenty-four years old. I asked him if this was around the time his addictions began. He looked startled, as if this was the first time anyone had asked the question. He replied, "Jack was my best friend and drinking buddy in university. We did everything together." I let the silence linger awhile. He lowered his head and began to sob. I referred him to a Jungian psychologist who specialized in treating addictions. He made excellent progress and recovery.

DOG STINKHORN
(Mutinus elegans)

INDICATIONS: womb, money, circumcision, control, gender identity, corporate, empathy, hero's journey, obsession

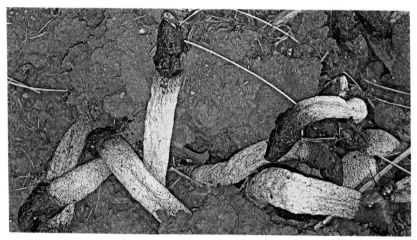

Dog stinkhorn (*Mutinus elegans* [Montagne] E. Fischer)

A man is measured by the expanse of the
moral horizon he chooses to inhabit.
—SANDOR MCNAB

Corporation: An ingenious device for obtaining
profit without individual responsibility.
—AMBROSE BIERCE

Manhood coerced into sensitivity is no manhood at all.
—CAMILLE PAGLIA

Sometimes, if you wear suits for too long, it changes your ideology.
—JOE SLOVO

The revolution that freed women from stereotypical pathways has led to a great deal of uncertainty and confusion over what it means to be male in modern society. Keen guides us in helping understand the issues:

> *The average man spends a lifetime denying, defending against, trying to control and reacting to the power of WOMAN. He is committed to remaining unconscious and out of touch with his own deepest feelings and experience.... We begin to learn the mysteries unique to maleness only when we separate from WOMAN'S world. But before we can take our leave we must first become conscious of the ways in which we are enmeshed, incorporated, inwombed, and defined by WOMAN. Otherwise we will be controlled by what we haven't remembered.*[2]

Circumcision is done today for cultural or religious reasons. It should be the owner of the penis who decides how he would like it to look and function, but that choice is rarely considered. The procedure removes about fifteen square inches of skin containing twenty thousand nerves (in adults). This does affect sexual sensitivity.

Female genital mutilation is common in twenty-seven countries and may involve more than 133 million women. This is a serious concern, but is not addressed by this mushroom essence.

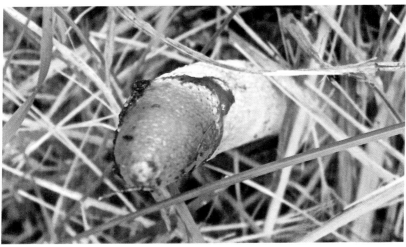

Dog stinkhorn

Essence description

Dog stinkhorn mushroom essence is for men seeking to connect with ideals of strength, passion, and meaning.

Dog stinkhorn essence can help ease the loss and anger associated with the primitive and brutal rite of circumcision. This barbaric practice was a sacrament that helped early societies create a social body— the tribe—at the sacrifice of individualization. This early wound gave a message to males that masculinity requires a wounding of the body. Manhood is thus achieved by our willingness to be mutilated by elders. The securing of gender identity helped maintain boundaries and manners between the sexes. Tribal societies focused on the past as a way to remain loyal to their ancestors' view of the world. Keen continues to enlighten us:

> *For reasons that are far from obvious, men's egos are nearly inseparable from their penises ... that is why sex is so important for us. A woman once told me, "I finally understood that for most men the penis is their only 'feminine' part. It is only when they are doing things with it that they allow themselves to feel." ... But if WOMAN is the promise of paradise, she is also the place of judgment and the entrance to hell. Since our entrance to the earthly paradise depends on her good graces, we give her the power to judge and reward or punish us ... we try to please her. But whether we enter into sex in the mood of sport-fucking or in tender relationship, we will be disappointed if we expect to find the proof of our masculinity there. Sex may bring pleasure or joy, but not identity.... It takes a very secure person to surrender to another in love.[3]*

Today, modern man is seeking a new way of being. The poet Robert Bly suggests we have raised a whole generation of sensitive men lacking thunder and lightning, the very elements bringing mushroom fruiting bodies to the surface of the earth.

Men have been trained to journey into the masculine womb, the corporation. Climbing the economic ladder has replaced the hero's journey in order to discover the heights and depths of the human psyche. It has become honorable, in the economic myth, to do whatever it takes to make a living. Men put aside their dreams and begin to dress and tailor themselves for the market. The ritual of wearing a suit and securing a tie around the neck suggests compliance with this form of emasculation. Moore explains:

Money is like sex. Some people believe that the more sexual experiences they have, with as many different people as possible, the more fulfilled they will be. But even great quantities of money and sex may not satisfy the craving. The problem lies not in having too much or too little, but in taking money literally, as a fetish rather than as a medium.... Like sex, money is so numinous, so filled with fantasy and emotion and resistant to rational guidance, that although it has much to offer, it can easily swamp the soul and carry consciousness off into compulsion and obsession.[4]

Female executives, despite the hidden belief of feminists, have not changed the rules of business, nor have they brought love and human kindness to the boardroom.

Dog stinkhorn mushroom essence helps males develop their reconnection with empathy. The healthy male, when met, is obvious to all. They give other people permission to be themselves. They do not view relationships in terms of position or stature. They develop and nurture friendships with men and women alike. They value self-exploration and personal, altruistic growth. They possess soul connection, and it is obvious to all around them.

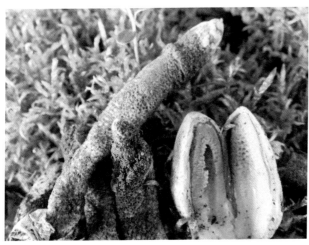

Dog stinkhorn

PREPARATION: This mushroom essence is prepared from fruiting bodies in rainwater under four hours of direct moonlight. Ideally, prepare the essence in solar and lunar phases of Leo or Taurus, during the full moon. Preserve the water one-to-one with brandy.

CASE STUDY: Dave was thirty-five years old, married seventeen years, with two children. He worked as an assistant manager of a sporting goods department in a large chain store. The client presented himself very well-dressed and manicured, with a soft handshake. He was concerned because he was suffering erectile dysfunction. We explored the issue further and found that early in his married life, with the first woman with whom he had sex, he experienced premature ejaculation. He had been circumcised shortly after birth. He admitted their love life was suffering. His wife had a full-time job, and they were raising two children that required transportation to hockey, soccer, swimming, and ballet. He said, "I no longer feel like a man." I suggested that he had not been able to complete the transition from adolescent to mature male. He was unsure what I meant, but just nodded. I suggested he try dog stinkhorn mushroom essence for a lunar cycle. I showed him the picture above and he joked that it reminded him of his erectile condition. He agreed to try it.

He returned in two months and was a changed man. He shook my hand firmly and informed me he had quit his job. While taking the drops he found himself suffering more irritation at work, and came to the realization that ten more years of this day-to-day boredom might lead to a promotion to department manager. "I realized I wanted more out of life," he said. I asked about his issue with impotence. He said he went home, told his wife he had quit work, and took her straight to the bedroom. "It was our best sex in ten years," he said.

BIRD'S NEST •
STRIATED BIRD'S NEST

(Cyathus striatus)

INDICATIONS: lucid dreaming, flying

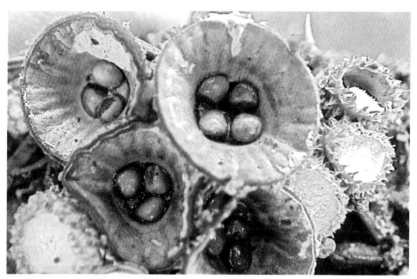

Bird's nest (*Cyathus striatus* [Hudson] Wildenow)

Who looks outside, dreams; who looks inside, awakes.

—CARL JUNG

Birds born in cages think that flying is a disease.

—ALEJANDRO JODOROWSKY

Your soul dreams those dreams. Not your body. Not your mind. The soul travels all over the world when you dream.

—JOHN THUNDERBIRD, CHIPPEWA ELDER

Lucid dreams can bring a personal sense of power and freedom. The experience is as if we are awake, and can help us achieve higher levels of awareness. There is a sequence of events, not usual in most dreaming, in which we can interact with other realities. The connection is this: flying dreams are a lower level of projections of consciousness. If we are able to take control of the experience, it suggests great lucidity and a high level of consciousness.

Recent studies have found that a region of the brain involved in self-reflection is larger in lucid dreamers. It is linked to metacognition, that is, thinking about thinking. Frequent lucid dreamers have a greater volume anterior prefrontal cortex. It is involved in conscious cognitive processes and plays a role in our ability to self-reflect.[5] This is not a statement of judgment but an observation of how dream states can influence waking consciousness and how day-to-day awareness can help shape our dreams.

Have you ever experienced a life-and-death scenario? If so, remember back to how the hours and days after a brush with death helped sweeten and lighten the following moments. How you savored being alive and fully soul-connected. Bird's nest mushroom essence helps bring renewed sweetness to life in a childlike manner. It reestablishes soul connection by reducing automatic response and seeing each new experience through the eyes of a child and the heart of a fully self-actualized mature being.

Native Americans believe we have three souls: ego soul associated with breath, body soul associated with life force, and free soul that leaves the body during dreams.

Essence description

Bird's nest mushroom essence relates to issues around dreaming, and lucid dreaming in particular. Lucid dreams occur when we become aware that we are dreaming and can direct our inner journey. Often flying dreams are included in this process.

The mushroom essence may be valuable in several ways. The first is by helping us experience our first lucid or flying dream. This is a new experience for many people, and the essence will help make the transition more comfortable, and at the same time more colorful.

In lucid dreaming, we control our choices and dictate internal experience. Ask to be taken where you will. Do not change dream characters but enter into dialogue with them inside the dream. Take the mushroom essence before sleep to help this process.

PREPARATION: Bird's nest mushroom essence is prepared by dropping rainwater into a number of the nests. Allow the water to sit in the nests for three or four nights around the full moon. This is removed with a pipette and combined with equal parts of brandy.

CASE STUDY 1: Tania was twenty-four years old, single, and a full-time legal assistant. She came to me as a client with an unusual request. She was told by her girlfriend that I worked with mushroom essences and that they might help her dream. I replied that everyone dreams, but it takes attention to remember them. She wanted to try the mushroom essence, so I suggested a lunar cycle with the proviso she kept a dream journal. She agreed.

She returned in four weeks with her journal. The writing started out sparse during the first ten days and then was filled with all kinds of dreams, including lucid and flying experiences. She was very pleased.

CASE STUDY 2: Nathan was a forty-two-year-old high school teacher. He was single and lived with his widowed mother. He had a very successful and rewarding career. He came to see me about a recurring dream. I asked him if he dreamed often, and he replied he did not remember any dreams except this one, about his father, that appeared occasionally over the past decade. I suggested bird's nest mushroom essence for a lunar cycle and that he keep a dream journal.

He came in one month later and was quite shaken and upset. He took the essence as directed and had several nights of disturbed sleep. One night, about ten days into the cycle, he dreamed that he was flying alongside his deceased father. It disturbed him so much he stopped taking the essence. We talked about his father, and how much he missed him. He had died of pancreatic cancer when Nathan was only eighteen years old. I suggested he begin to take the mushroom essence again, and if his father appeared, to engage him in conversation. He was uncertain that would happen, but agreed.

Three weeks later, he came to see me, and he appeared very different. He said he met his father, and they flew and talked in one dream. His father asked him why he was still single, and Nathan reminded him that on his deathbed he had been asked to take care of his mother. Immediately, his father turned into a raven and flew off. "What does it mean?" asked Nathan. I asked him if he ever desired to have his own life, and move out of his mother's home. He confessed that he wanted to, but felt guilty even thinking about it. I suggested he talk to his mother about it.

He phoned me two days later. He had talked to her, and she told him it was about time he moved out; she was worried about him getting on with his life. Everything changed.

WESTERN GIANT PUFFBALL
(Calvatia booniana)

INDICATIONS: sin; aggression; obsessive-compulsive disorder; anal, genital, and oral fixations; anxiety; masturbation; competition; mooning; pornography; destruction; frustration; receptivity

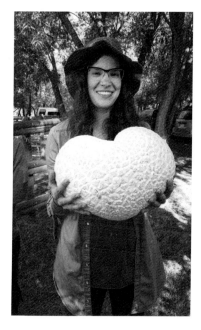

Robert's student Desiree Serna Klassen
Western giant puffball
(*Calvatia booniana* A. H. Smith)

Where talent is a dwarf, self-esteem is a giant.
—JEAN ANTOINE PETIT-SENN

Philosophy is to the real world as masturbation is to sex.
—KARL MARX

Give me masturbation or give me death.
—HOMER, ILIAD 2

The four principal activities through which we form ego are oral, anal, urethral, and genital. The necessary states for ego development cannot be skipped or repressed, and this all begins early in life. The significance of each stage needs to be consciously examined and its meaning incorporated when issues of imbalance are limiting connection with soul. Whitmont explains:

> *Orally, we grasp into ourselves. Anally, we hold and force out substance, formed matter; we prevail, we establish our own impulse expressions where automatic life manifestations are concerned. Urethrally, we pour forth, give and create, or we restrain and control ourselves. Genitally, we arouse ourselves and enter into union with the "other."*[6]

Due to early childhood trauma, there may be distortion of physical as well as mental and emotional health related to these specific organ systems.

Essence description

Giant puffball fungal essence relates to the development of ego and its relationship to bodily functions. Giant puffball essence helps individuals move through the stages of preoccupation with erotic parts of the body. The oral stage, represented by sucking, drinking, and kissing, expresses receptivity and yielding. Any distortion of this early dependent reaction can lead to frustration. Biting, for example, expresses clinging, grasping, and greed. Giant puffball essence may help issues associated with this stage, including lack of comfort from breast-feeding. Nail biting is one manifestation of this inner lack of comfort. Obsession with large breasts, milk production, and needs to suckle are related to this stage.

The anal phase was referred to as the sadistic phase by Freud and associated with aggression and self-assertion. There is an unconscious desire to turn an automatic response of the intestines into an accomplishment and increased independence. The control of defecation provides young children with a sense of power to gratify their physical needs.

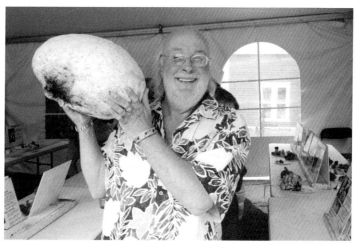

Robert with a giant puffball at the Telluride Mushroom Festival

Early potty-training and trauma around this issue can create lifelong issues. It is an expression of egotism, but also the necessity to strive for ego.

Exposing the buttocks, known as mooning, is typically a masculine pursuit reflecting ego assertion against the feminine. It was a popular expression for a generation feeling threatened by modern-day depersonalized conformity and herd mentality. It is an outward expression of fear associated with owning our own feminine. Anxiety surrounding power, competition, and destructiveness is triggered in this phase.

Giant puffball mushroom essence may assist many issues surrounding discipline and the various shadows of associated repression. The anal-retentive personality is one example of stagnation or blockage of ego development at this stage. As a reaction to early or harsh toilet training, the young child may hold back in rebellion. This later forms an adult who hates a mess, is obsessively tidy and punctual, and respects authority. They may also be somewhat stubborn and very prudent with finances. The anal character exhibits eight diagnostic features of obsessive-compulsive personality disorder (OCPD). Coprolalia (shit speech) is a prominent feature of Tourette's syndrome. Giant puffball and snake liverwort essences may help modify or curb this scatological distortion. Irritable bowel syndrome, for example, is associated with a high level of neuroticism, problems with self-assertion, and reported history of abuse.

Urination represents yielding or controlling an outgoing libido stream. According to Whitmont: "The ego learns to choose between allowing the outpouring to pass or withholding it…. The urge and its restraint form the instinctual basis for an identity which one experiences in giving, in becoming master of oneself, a morally disciplined 'pure' person."[7] Repeated bladder infections, especially in those sexually abused, may find relief from this mushroom essence, by bringing to awareness the original "insult" and pain. Imbalance, such as the need for participating in "golden showers," is addressed. The expression *pissed-off* relates to a heated, inflamed condition. Late training in children has been linked to urinary incontinence and infections.

The genital stage relates to initial self-arousal and masturbation. It is the final stage of creating "I," and the original primitive magical all-identity is overcome. Whitmont notes, "Masturbation expresses the final point of transition from narcissistic nondualistic participation to the relative freedom of dualistic consciousness."[8] Distortion at this level may lead young girls to wish to be boys, or "penis envy," later turning into desire for her father by substituting this wish with desire to have a baby. This is often associated with tension between mother and daughter.

This mushroom essence combines well with shaggy mane for obsessive-compulsive activity associated with pornography. Distortions at various anxiety levels, such as fear of self-exploration, judgment and sin, or compulsive and obsessive needs are diminished. An ability to foretell the future may increase. A tendency to possess or develop thick skin may be resolved. This includes physical skin conditions such as scleroderma and formation of keloid scar tissue. Add a few drops of the essence to distilled water and spritz the affected areas twice daily.

It may combine well with cinnabar, snake liverwort, or velvet foot mushroom essences for various skin conditions. The underlying patterns will suggest the proper combination.

PREPARATION: Western giant puffball essence is produced by covering the surface of rainwater in a crystal bowl with a complete layer of spores for one hour during the waxing of the moon.

CASE STUDY 1: Anne was thirty-seven years old, married, with no children, operating her own retail business. She came to me complaining

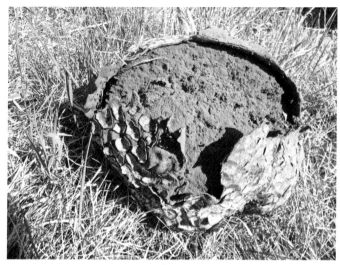

Millions of spores from a giant puffball

of constipation and chronic urethritis and cystitis (bladder infections). She had suffered bladder problems since the age of thirteen and had been on courses of antibiotics and cranberry juice for over twenty years. The condition was aggravated by sex, with increasing levels of frustration for both her and her partner. A quick urinalysis found she had been treating the physical condition incorrectly. Her urine, when infected, was acidic, and cranberry juice was not helping. We chose an herbal formula that gave her more than symptomatic relief so she did not have to take more antibiotics. We then delved into the deeper issue—her need for control. She strongly denied this was a problem, but consented to give giant puffball mushroom essence a trial for one lunar cycle. She was asked to keep a dream journal.

Four weeks later she returned with an apprehensive look on her face. She had a dream in which she remembered herself masturbating at age thirteen and experiencing her first orgasm. She soaked the bed with ejaculate, but thought she had wet the bed with urine. Her bladder infections began soon afterward. I suggested a possible link and referred her to a Jungian psychologist. Conscious awareness of the link between psychosomatic urogenital imbalance, letting go, and ego development helped resolve her long-standing issue.

CASE STUDY 2: Karl was a fifty-three-year-old Roman Catholic priest. He came to me suffering with chronic prostatitis. It was a recurring problem for nearly twenty years, temporarily cleared up with antibiotics. I asked the obvious question of frequency of masturbation. He became very angry, but he was controlled and hid it well. I suggested that it was normal and healthy to frequently empty this gland. He did not reply. I suggested western giant puffball mushroom essence for a lunar cycle, and he reluctantly agreed. I really did not expect to see him again.

A month later, he returned, sat down, and apologized. I asked, "For what?" He replied, "You hit a nerve when you asked me about my sex life, because we are supposed to be above our carnal urges." I told him that I did not mean any offense or embarrassment, and he stopped me. "I took the essence, and three nights later, I had a nocturnal emission. It frightened me, and I felt guilty, but I did rather enjoy it." He then confided that he had been relieving himself twice a week lately, and felt fine with it. Two years later, he reported there had been no recurrence of his prostate issue.

JELLY FUNGUS •
YELLOW WITCH'S BUTTER

(Tremella mesenterica)

INDICATIONS: envy, jealousy, paranoia, illusion, misery, flexibility, wisdom

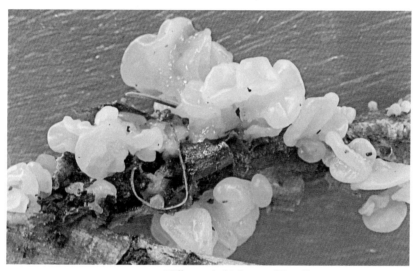

Yellow witch's butter (*Tremella mesenterica* Retzius)

Do not overrate what you have received, nor envy others.
He who envies others does not obtain peace of mind.
—BUDDHA

Jealousy is both reasonable and belongs to reasonable men,
while envy is base and belongs to the base, for the one
makes himself good things by jealousy, while the other does
not allow his neighbor to have them through envy.
—ARISTOTLE

Hatred is active, and envy passive dislike; there
is but one step from envy to hate.
—GOETHE

Yellow witch's butter mushroom essence is related to envy and its ugly cousin, jealousy. Envy and jealousy share much in common, but are entirely different feelings. Moore writes:

> One is a desire for what another person has, the other fear that the other person will take what we have, but they both have a corrosive effect on the heart. Either emotion can make a person feel ugly. There is nothing noble in either of them. At the same time, a person may feel oddly attached to them. The jealous person takes some pleasure in his suspicions, and the envious person feeds on his desire for what others possess.[1]

Yellow witch's butter mushroom essence helps us to understand the archetypal aspects of these emotions. It helps us realize the only path out of jealousy is through it. That is, we require the emotional pain associated with the wound in order to reexamine our mis-take. In theater, a scripted scene is acted out, and if there is a stumble or a correction, it is termed a "mis-take." This helps put our learning curve of life into perspective. We need to experience the feeling on a deep, soulful level in order to explore new territory and let go of the old and familiar patterns. Moore continues:

> Jealousy draws out a strange cast of characters—the moralist, the detective, the paranoid, the archconservative. The word paranoia is usually taken etymologically to mean knowledge (noia) that is "alongside" (para)—to be beside oneself, mad. But I prefer to think of it as knowledge that lies outside yourself.[2]

Think of those times in your own life when you wanted to share something amazing. And remember how often you were met with indifference or even hostility? Often, the people surrounding us are not aware of their reactions or how they may influence our own fragile psyche. George Orwell remarked, "the essence of being human is that one does not seek perfection."[3] Jealous ego and envy may start with sibling rivalry and manifest throughout your life. Moore concludes,

> These soul figures who pretend to know so much—the moralist and the rest—want to find out what is going on. They assume

that something is threatening and dangerous is afoot.... Paranoid knowing satisfies the masochist who takes delight in being hurt.... Paradoxically, if he were to allow his jealousy to work from within like a detective, on behalf of his soul, instead of as a free-wheeling paranoid complex, he would discover many things about himself and about love.... The paranoid element in his jealousy both keeps the possibility of deeper knowledge within reach but also dissociates itself from will and intentionality. It remains unrealistic and twisted, and yet it is the raw material for wisdom.[4]

There is no skipping of steps when it comes to soul connection.

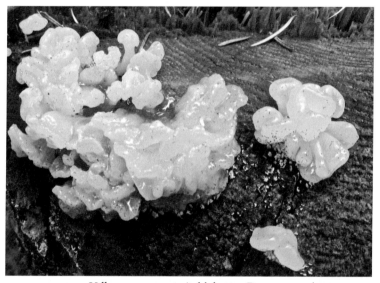

Yellow or orange witch's butter *Dacrymyces palmatus* grows
on conifers, and *Tremella mesenterica* on hardwood.

Essence description

Yellow witch's butter essence helps us to better understand past and present encounters with the archetypal patterns of envy and jealousy and help release their hold on our psyche.

Envy is one of the seven deadly sins. At first glance, it looks like an ego issue but is in fact a soul issue. The ego problem is how to react to envy, and then figure out what the heart actually desires.

We may feel that we are victims of fate or character, that we have been cheated or deprived. Counseling and positive affirmations will not work. It may be best to allow ourselves to feel the emptiness deeply, to understand this feeling from the depths of our soul. Yellow witch's butter mushroom essence will assist the sometimes painful journey to the underworld and soul connection.

Both jealousy and envy are fantasies of illusion. Moore explains:

> But dwelling in an imaginary life is a way of avoiding soul. Soul is always attached to life in some way. As symptoms, jealousy and envy keep life at a safe distance; as invitations to soul, they both offer ways into one's own heart where love and attachment can be reclaimed. The fact that jealousy and envy are both resistant to reason and to human efforts to eradicate them is a blessing. They ask us for a deeper diving into the soul, beyond ideas of health and happiness and into mystery.[5]

Yellow witch's butter mushroom essence helps release us from the need to fix something and rather get on with our lives and stop repressing our experiences of jealousy and envy. The essence helps us feel and experience our emotions, observe our reactions, and then connect with soul wounds. Only then can true healing begin.

Stirring the witch's mythical cauldron, and stewing in the messy juices of misery, help us transform our lives into greater riches of depth, maturity, and flexibility.

PREPARATION: Yellow Witch's Butter essence is prepared from fresh fruiting bodies in rainwater contained in a crystal bowl. This is best done when the moon is in Scorpio.

CASE STUDY: Chelsea was twenty-two, single, and having an affair with an older married man. She came to see if I could help with her long-standing and persistent chlamydia infection. Three bouts of antibiotics had not addressed the problem. We used a protocol of the essential oil *Thymus vulgaris* var. *thujanol* that I learned about from a medical aromatherapist from France.

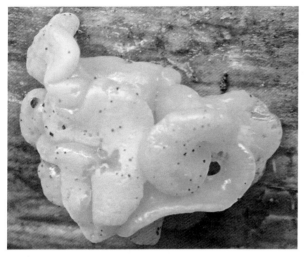

Yellow witch's butter

This oral, vaginal, and rectal therapy helped clear her body of this persistent pathogen in about three weeks. At her next visit she thanked me and then confided she was feeling jealous of her lover's wife. We started to explore this simple, yet complex, issue. I suggested she take yellow witch's butter mushroom essence for a lunar cycle, and to keep a dream journal. She returned four weeks later, smiling and looking very relieved.

Sixteen days after starting to take the mushroom essence, she felt the need to confront her lover about him leaving his wife. He said he wanted to, and she could feel him lying as he said it. That night, she had a dream of sleuthing with the fictional character Nancy Drew on a detective adventure. They were hired by a woman who believed her husband was cheating, and she wanted photographic proof of his affair. She awoke startled, and realized her feelings of envy and jealousy were of her own making. I asked her how it would feel to be his wife, and she replied that she had already decided and had told him the affair was over.

NOTE: Nancy Drew is a fictional young girl detective series, first appearing in 1930. In 2004, the original Nancy Drew Mystery Stories ended and Girl Detectives was launched. Feminist literary critics suggest she is variously a mythic hero, an expression of wish fulfillment, or an embodiment of contradictory ideas about femininity.

WOOD EAR
(Auricularia auricula)

INDICATIONS: auditory hallucinations, silence, inner voice, doors of perception, listening, tinnitus, Ménière's disease, stillness, autism spectrum disorder, verbal communication

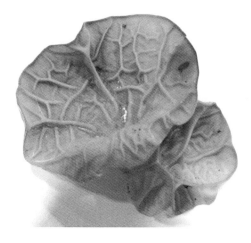

Wood ear
(Auricularia auricula
[L.] Underwood)

He that hath ears to hear, let him hear.
—MATTHEW 11:15

Much silence has a mighty noise.
—SWAHILI PROVERB

The soul has been given its own ears to hear
things that the mind does not understand
—RUMI

Many people possess an inner voice that speaks to them during times of decision-making. It is an external amplification of inner thought. The *Iliad,* one of the great epics of classical Greek literature, is filled with voice-hearing, usually from gods living on the Pantheon. Herodotus wrote, "Men trust their ears less than their eyes."[6] Epimendes wrote about trances and conversation with spirits in the sixth century BCE. The Bible is rich in calls from heavenly voices. Moses, Joan of Arc, Socrates, Martin Luther, William Blake, and President George W. Bush all experienced voice-hearing and shared it with the world. Blake wrote, "For man has closed himself up, till he sees thro' narrow chinks of his cavern."[7]

Today, in the biomedical model, voice-hearing is considered a sign of mental illness and a symptom of schizophrenia. In rural India, ringing in the ears is believed to be of divine origin. Yet one study of 15,000 people from Baltimore found over 2,000 individuals reported hearing voices. It is not that unusual. Between 30 million and 50 million Americans suffer various degrees of tinnitus.

Stephen Buhner contributes from his book *Plant Intelligence and the Imaginal Realm:*

> *This is, in fact, what many schizophrenics and those on hallucinogens experience—and it happens for a specific reason that is most definitely not pathological. It is crucial to our habitation of this planet and this book is about, in part, learning to open sensory channels at will to whatever degree is desired—to open the doors of perception.[8]*

The concept of sensory gating channels allows us to focus attention on what is important and what needs to be filtered out, protecting us from sensory overload. It helps us distinguish self from nonself.

Transcendental or Buddhist meditation, yoga, and other mental disciplines utilize quieting of the mind to bring calmness and serenity to the psyche and spirit. A mantra is often utilized in the former, so that the repetition of a rhythmic sound will shut out extraneous chatter and allow us to experience stillness. This process helps to strengthen our will and connection with soul.

In the Chinese tradition, the eye represents yang sense and expresses the sun. The ear represents yin sense and embodies the moon. In fact, the ear is shaped like an embryo. Berendt writes that our ear is assimilating, receptive, passive, and feminine.[9] He notes the moon vibrates at 422 hertz and is associated with G sharp, which is not commonly used today, but in the past was associated with the tuning forks of Mozart, Handel, and Bach.

One method that I have found most useful for creating a space of silence in our modern world is flotation chambers. Filled with salt water at body temperature (94.5 degrees Fahrenheit), the dark chamber allows us to experience the sounds of our own body.

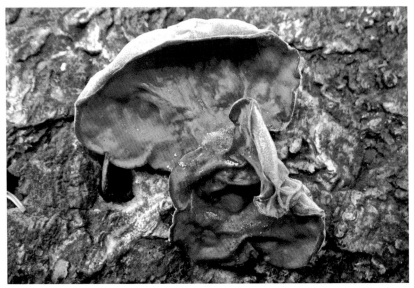

Wood ear

Essence description

Wood Ear mushroom essence assists those individuals who experience voice-hearing or what are called auditory hallucinations.

Tinnitus and Ménière's disease may be relieved with wood ear mushroom essence. These two distinctly different conditions may be projected and treated as physiological by biomedicine, but there are often distinct, and yet related, deep-seated mental and emotional patterns. Tinnitus is a reminder to listen to what is being said, or to listen more closely to our own voice. In some cultures, ringing in the ears means our soul is crying. Ménière's disease is about finding more balance in life. Sometimes there is an unwillingness to hear something, or someone. Increasing narrow-mindedness may be present. Wood ear mushroom essence helps us listen to our body and accept information from various cellular levels regarding health or discomfort.

Verbal and nonverbal autism spectrum disorder may be helped with wood ear mushroom essence and luminescent Panellus.

Wood ear mushroom essence helps us to discern whether our inner voice is coming from a place of balance or fear. The latter can result in paranoia or patterns of misguided projections onto others. Note the similarity of the words *fear, hear, ear, bear, tear, dear, near, year* and *wear.* In disassociated states, there can be confusion and inaccurate intake of communication. In states of imbalance, words may be spoken, or decisions made, that cannot easily be taken back.

Sacred speech and silence nurture the soul, but constant superficial chatter interferes with tuning into the frequency of soul connection. Observe the difference.

PREPARATION: Wood ear essence is produced in a crystal bowl containing rainwater around the full moon, or when the lunar orb is in the sign of Libra.

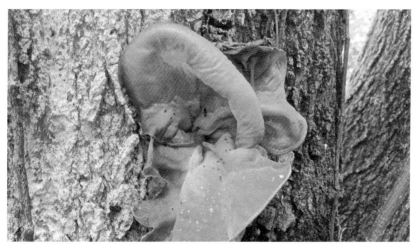

Wood ear

CASE STUDY: Phil was forty-four years old, married, with one child, working in sales for a large printing firm. He came to see me concerning noises in his ears. The first noises started about three years earlier, and at first were high-pitched sounds of short duration, followed by crackling and bubbling sensations. Tests by various medical doctors and hearing specialists revealed no pathological concern. Recently, however, the noise changed to voices with intermittent sounds, like a muted talk show on the radio. This was deeply disconcerting, as his recently deceased mother had been diagnosed as schizophrenic and was on medication for many years. I suggested he take wood ear mushroom essence for a lunar cycle and keep a dream journal.

When he returned, he suggested that nothing had happened, that the voices were still there. I carefully looked over his journal writing and noted one passage: "July 18th. Fell asleep and had a dream of an angel blowing a trumpet." I asked him what that might mean. Who was the angel, and what did the trumpet represent? Unraveling this dream took over three hours. He had felt abandoned by his mother, and help-less to make her feel better when she was alive. He began to cry, and this continued for a long period of time. The noises did not return.

PEZIZA
(Peziza badia)

INDICATIONS: chaos, cleanliness, control, love, neuroses, detachment, paranoia

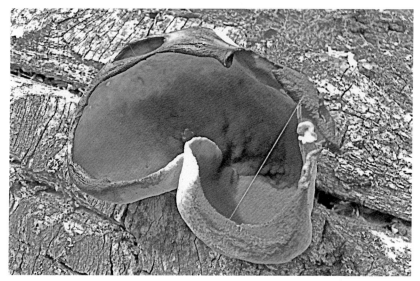

Peziza (*Peziza badia* Persoon)

Just because you are paranoid does not mean there's nobody after you.
—OLD SAYING

If the national mental illness of the United States is megalomania, that of Canada is paranoid schizophrenia.
—MARGARET ATWOOD

Cleanliness is almost as bad as godliness.
—H. L. MENCKEN

Striving for perfection is well-intentioned and understandable. It is an attempt to control our inner fragmentation and disconnection from soul, and to help create meaning in life. However, it can easily lead to neuroses and even paranoia, if carried to an extreme.

The early philosopher Empedocles noted that if the world was perfect, it could not improve, and thus lacked "true perfection," which depends on progress. Aristotle believed *perfect* meant "complete," as in nothing to add or subtract. In *Metaphysics*, he gives two other meanings of the term: one is that something is so good, nothing of the kind could be better; and the other is that which has attained its purpose.

If we are perfect and complete, how do we allow for the concept or the reality of being loved? K. M. Abenheimer puts it well:

> *The paranoiac, for instance, is obsessed by his longing to be loved. He has rejected the dirty chthonian (underground) power in himself as well as outside and tries to be perfect and deserving of love. Yet he has lost hope of finding reliable love. Therefore his demanding dependent side has to be suppressed too, and he lives by the controlling pure will only.*[1]

Note the reference to underground. "Chthonian" is from the Greek *khthonios,* meaning "under the earth." This relates to soul work, the nitty-gritty process of achieving shadow awareness.

Essence description

Peziza mushroom essence relates to those individuals who find aspects of earthly existence "dirty" or "unclean," or individuals who are detached or ungrounded. They seek perfection in their own lives and believe they can create a perfect world through controlling their environment. Recent research suggests that increases in childhood asthma are related to our clean environments, and that dirt, disease, and death are interlinked in a complex immune cycle of function.

The oyster creates a beautiful pearl, but only with the presence of an irritating grain of sand. Shamans smoke a cigarette after an intense entheogenic journey to come back to the world of others. This desire for perfection requires immense mental effort that invariably gives way

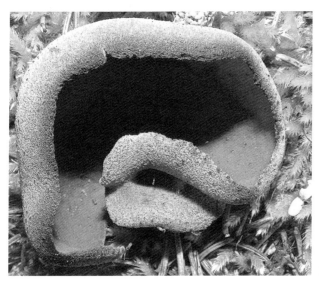

Peziza

to chaos, lack of control, and fragmentation. It may relate to aspects of perfection and combines well with giant puffball mushroom essence.

Paranoia may result from the attempt to control something we cannot control. It combines well with yellow witch's butter in some situations.

The earth element is often lacking in some individual's natal charts, further exasperating this imbalance. A medical astrologer may be a useful referral in such cases. Activities such as hiking in the woods, camping, taking up pottery, nature photography, walking barefoot, and picking edible and medicinal mushrooms will help ground us. Connection to nature and wilderness helps us discover the quality of our own soul.

You do not have to be a professional astrologer to understand the energetic imbalance present in a client's chart. Earth, air, water, and fire work in balance. A lack of the air element would suggest the client do breath work; a lack of water may be balanced with learning to swim or living by a body of water. An excess of fire may suggest encouraging the client to stop smoking, or reduce their intake of fried foods and add more raw fruits and vegetables. You get the idea.

Peziza essence works best when combined with an affirmation. You can create your own, including reference to being present here and now, stable and secure.

I have found Peziza mushroom essence and Crab Apple from the English Flower Essences of Dr. Bach are very synergistic. The connection of soul and spirit addresses issues of perfection simultaneously.

PREPARATION: This mushroom essence is produced by placing rainwater into cupped, living fruiting bodies, overnight, during a Virgo moon. Pipette the water in the morning and combine with equal parts of brandy.

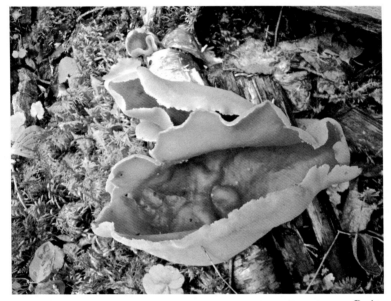

Peziza

CASE STUDY: Stephanie was thirty-nine years old, married, with one child. She came to my clinic for help with her constant abdominal pain. She was dressed simply, but everything matched perfectly: hair, nails, and skin were all hygienic and perfect. Lipstick and nail color were identical. Whole batteries of medical tests could not find any pathology that would explain her constant gripping and debilitating pain. While sitting in the chair opposite mine, she began to move objects on my desk into symmetrical alignment.

We talked about her life a little more, and then she took a tissue from the box on my desk and started to "dust" my slit lamp microscope

I use for iridology. I asked her if she considered cleaning her own home very important. She became very defensive, her nose turned up, and her lip curled. "Of course, doesn't anyone with any self-respect?" she replied. I suggested that she may be trying too hard to control all aspects of life, and she sighed and admitted it was a lot of work to keep things "running perfectly." I suggested she take Peziza mushroom essence for a lunar cycle to see if it would help her abdominal issue. She agreed.

One month later, she appeared in my office with an entirely different appearance. She apologized for her casual dress, noting she had just come from a walk by the river with her dog. I asked about the dog, and she confirmed that two weeks ago, their daughter was transferred for work and could no longer care for Dusty, her golden retriever. I asked if the dog lived indoors, and she said, "I know she's messy, but she's such good company." At the end of session I asked about the abdominal pain. She thanked me for the mushroom remedy and noted that after the first two weeks, it just went away.

GREEN ELF CUP

(Chlorociboria aeruginascens)

communication, compassion, heart, judgment, friendship

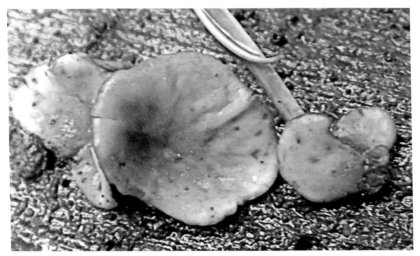

Green elf cup (*Chlorociboria aeruginascens* Karouse
ex C. S. Ramamurthi, Korf & L. R. Batra)

*A person suffers if he or she is constantly being forced into the
statistical mentality and away from the road of feeling.*

—ROBERT BLY

The essence of communication is intention.

—WERNER ERHARD

This turquoise-colored mushroom is sometimes found on rotting wood.
If we break into the log, we will expose a deep marine blue-colored
mycelium. It suggests a connection between the heart and throat chakras.

Western society puts great value on individuals who present their
ideas in a sequential, logical method, moving from 1 to 2 to 3 and so
on. This is frequently present in the mental patterns of those who see
the world in black and white. The strict adherence to dogmatic values

washes the color out of life. It creates a binary response to issues, creating simple reactions of right and wrong, or good and bad.

Judgment may become more important than humanity. Being right becomes more important than feelings from the heart and soul. Western philosophy is one of judgment, separation, and criticism, something we inherited from ancient Greeks such as Plato. Criticism derives from the Greek *krin* , meaning "sever," "divide," "separate," "select," "choose," or "prefer."

But there is another way to practice our true vocation. With heart-centered soul connection, it is possible to be successful in any chosen field of endeavor. Recent research suggests that all incoming information is processed for a millisecond through the heart before moving to the brain. Buhner touches on this subject:

> *The American awareness of heart field dynamics is incredibly stunted. To a large degree that is a consequence of the abandonment of feeling as a primary cognitive approach to the world. The substitution of a mind-only reasoning process based on linear reductionism—inoculated so strongly in the school system—results in a strong repression of both the use of the heart field and caring in general.[2]*

This is not to say rational thinking is not valuable, just highly overrated. Albert Einstein is quoted as saying "Imagination is more information than knowledge. For knowledge is limited to all we now know and understand, while imagination embraces the entire world, and all there ever will be to know and understand."[3]

Essence description

Green elf cup mushroom essence helps promote open communication and clear thinking. It may be useful when there is confusion around direction in life.

The mushroom essence may be helpful to teachers, authors, journalists, and television and radio personalities. It may combine well with shaggy mane for writer's block. The essence is not for promoting more linear or logical thinking, as we may suppose, but for helping us express our ideas and opinions in a more eloquent and emotive manner.

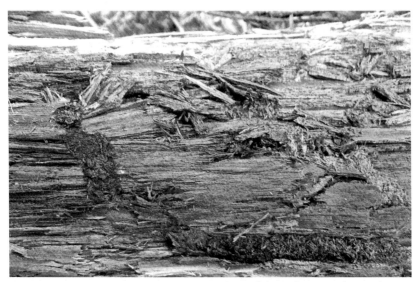

Green-stained wood that is home to the mushroom

Green elf cup mushroom essence helps those wishing to communicate with individuals who respond to linear concepts by helping move the discussion or argument through the heart. Green elf cup helps us attract long-lasting, soul-based friendships. It combines well with honey mushroom essence for this purpose. When communication is clear, and we are receptive to universal feedback, the gates of empathy, compassion, and caring swing wide open.

PREPARATION: The mushroom essence is prepared from fresh fruiting bodies laid on rainwater for one night in a crystal bowl, under a Cancer moon. The next day, equal parts of water and brandy are combined.

CASE STUDY: Josh was twenty-four years old, single, and writing his doctoral thesis in quantum physics. This brilliant young man came to my office complaining of insomnia, headaches, and tremors in his hands. I asked if he was feeling stressed, to which he nodded affirmatively. I suggested, after further inquiry, a nervine formula that would relax the body but still allow for mental acuity. Almost as an after-thought, I asked how the thesis was proceeding. He admitted to suffering writer's block and having difficulty articulating the abstract

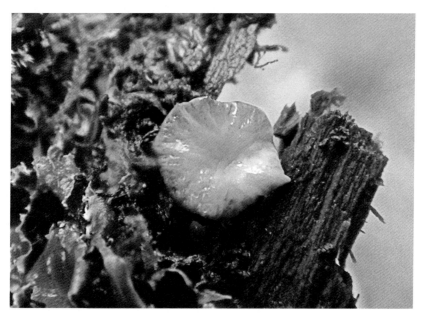

Insert caption here

patterns of his hypothesis into intelligent, linear thoughts. I suggested he try green elf cup mushroom essence for four weeks.

He returned and said he was not sure if it was the herbal formula or the mushroom essence that helped, but he was ecstatic about the rapid progress on his paper. "I had all of these fragments of information that required a framework. One night, I had a dream where everything reversed itself and turned upside down. I was walking through the jungle and snakes were consuming their tails and turning into amoeba. I touched one blobby creature, and it turned into a smiling dragon. It was pretty wild. I mean, my study is all about energy, but I never really thought about it from this perspective."

His writing became more fluid, and his physical symptoms disappeared.

BLACK MOREL

(Morchella snyderi)

INDICATIONS: DNA, fear, secrecy, projection, shadowboxing

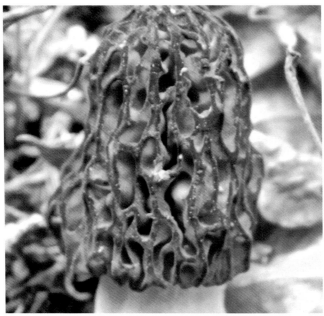

Morel (*Morchella snyderi* M. Kuo, Dewsbury,
Moncalvo & S. L. Stephenson)

In all chaos there is a cosmos, in all disorder a secret order.
—CARL JUNG

Truth never damages a cause that is just.
—MAHATMA GANDHI

*A culture of secrecy is like the bad stench created by
cat pee—it is very difficult to get rid of.*
—PIERRE DE VOS

Many people resist looking at parts of themselves for fear they will discover something terrible. They fear every thought or feeling, and attempt to hide it under their mental bed in the form of repression. They hold onto their inner fears in secret. Some individuals are so disconnected from this fear they cannot see it directly, but only as a reflection. Many people hide or deny this part of themselves, and thus forget their authentic self. They believe the person in the mirror is themselves, rather than the mask they have applied.

The spiritual teacher Lazaris said, "It is the shadow that hold the clues. The shadow also holds the secret of change, change that can affect you on a cellular level, change that can affect your very DNA."[4] By hiding and lying to ourselves, we deny ourselves the freedom to choose who we are and can become. By embracing our worst fears, we can become our greatest self.

This is why opposites attract. Couples will begin to cooperate like one person, with each trading strengths and weaknesses in compensation. A wise person once told me that men expect their female partners never to change, and they always do. And women have expectations that men can change, and they don't.

But this may only be true in relationships that do not work on evolving and growing into soul connection. Optimists attract pessimists, extroverts seek introverts, artists pursue scientists, and pragmatists enjoy the company of spiritual seekers. At some point in any relationship the traits that created attraction become the least attractive. And that is exactly why soul has brought these two individuals together. Without looking and examining our own shadow work, the process of shadowboxing is inevitable.

Essence description

Morel mushroom essence helps couples discover much deeper soul connection and move beyond the repetitive and painful exchanges associated with rejecting the other's disowned qualities. That is, the man who was initially attracted to the open, sexual woman may latter try to turn his partner into a mother figure, or she may become a sexless partner who is supposed to love him and display no shadow of her own.

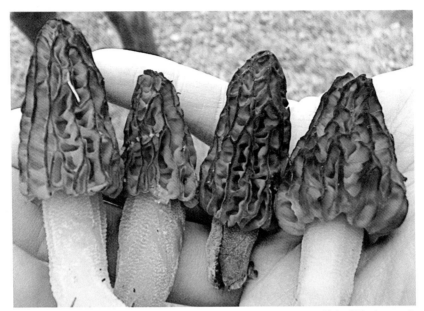

Handful of black morels

Or a woman may be attracted to a man who is optimistic, upbeat, and self-assured. In time, she desires more intimacy and finds his external, positive-all-the-time attitude intolerable. He may perceive this as an attempt to change him if he is far removed from his true authentic self.

Morel mushroom essence helps couples deal with what psychologists call projective identification. This is where one partner unconsciously identifies with the other's shadow and acts it out. This is where shadowboxing can arise.

James Hillman suggests we learn to love the negative shadow whenever it arises, to laugh at it, to care for it, and find ways to live with it.[5] Jung notes that the shadow appears as the same gender in night dreams to frighten or threaten our ego. The most important point is to pay attention to how our shadow projections affect others, and acknowledge them.[6]

Morel mushroom essence may be useful for couples that feel a sense of inequality in their relationship. This is the daemon on everyone's shoulder. A daemon or *daimōn,* from the ancient Greek tradition, represents the animal or divine spirit manifesting in your personality or soul. This was misinterpreted and written as "demon" in the Bible.

Morel mushroom essence will help establish connections based on the needs of soul, not the personality. By acknowledging the need to learn and differentiate between our desires of ego, soul, and shadow, we can come to a more deeply rewarding partnership of intimacy.

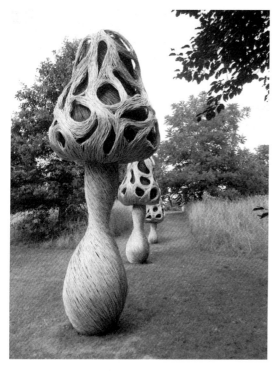

Willow woven morels in Kew Gardens, London, by artist Tom Hare (photo courtesy of Chanchal Cabrera)

PREPARATION: Morel essence is prepared by immersing the fresh fruiting bodies in rainwater in a crystal bowl overnight. Ideally this is done with full moon in Aquarius or Scorpio.

CASE STUDY: A couple, Carl, forty-five, and Nora, forty-three, were referred to me by a psychologist friend who specializes in marriage counseling. Carl works as bank manager, and Nora is a financial adviser with an insurance company. They were having ethical issues concerning another couple. One evening at a restaurant, they spotted their male friend having dinner with a woman they did not recognize. They were divided as to whether to tell his wife, not knowing the right course of action.

The secret became unbearable for Nora, and she told her friend, who in turn confronted her husband as to whether he was having an affair. He admitted that he was. This led in turn to a strong disagreement between Carl and Nora, and six months later, it festered and created a polarization of their relationship, which became frosty and uncomfortable. When they came to my office, this disagreement had been ongoing for nearly two years. I asked them to consider taking morel mushroom essence for a lunar cycle, and for each of them to keep a dream journal. She quickly consented, while he was reluctant and ambivalent.

Two weeks later, I received a phone call from their psychologist. She asked me what I had prescribed. I told her, and she let me know that significant progress happened in their last session. Nora started her financial career after their children went to university and was so successful she was making more than double her husband's salary. He was feeling insecure and finally admitted what was really bothering him.

OREGON WHITE TRUFFLE
(Tuber oregonense)

INDICATIONS: sexuality, romantic feelings, primal spark, shadow work, love, lust, imagination, boredom, discernment, freedom, equality, liberty, concealed development

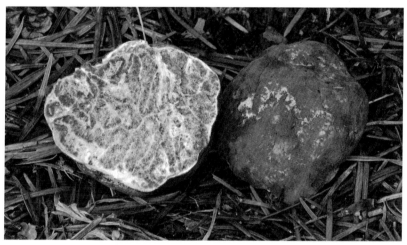

Oregon white truffle (*Tuber oregonense* Trappe, Bonito & Rawlinson)
(photo courtesy of Daniel Winkler)

We don't care to eat toadstools that think they are truffles.
—MARK TWAIN

You gotta have swine to show you where the truffles are.
—EDWARD ALBEE

Only a struggle twists sentimentality and lust together into love.
—E. M. FORSTER

Western civilization provides a degree of physical comfort never before realized on the planet. There also exists a plethora of external elements, involving excitation and distractions, with easy access to music, magazines, films, television, and the internet. Very seldom do these visitations lead to inspiration or inflame imagination. Rather, for many people they tend to be an escape from the boredom and monotony of our day-to-day lives. This is not always true, as great literature and music can uplift and increase connection with our higher self. It can lift the spirit and soothe the soul.

There is a dark side of human tendency to attack or ridicule individuals of fame or fortune when they fall from their pedestals. It is the herd mentality that enjoys the misfortune of others with higher social or financial standing. What is the root of such negativity? It is the shadow side of freedom, liberty, and equality. The shadow is what is true about us that we don't know. It is not a part of us we are aware of that we keep hidden or suppressed. The shadow is what our psyches repress, not what our egos suppress. Big difference.

There is a big difference between ego-based romance and soulful romance. Plotkin writes, "And yet romance is also the realm where we unleash our grandest and most delusional projections, where the shadow is sure to emerge in all its dark glory ... through its extreme currents and emotions, romance destabilizes the ego and opens a door to soul."[7]

When entering my astrological Saturn return around age twenty-seven, I married, divorced, and my house burned down (up?), within a short period of time. That is an example of soul-driven opportunity for change. Out of the ashes rises increased awareness. We see the partner or ourselves as flawed, but often refuse to reject the projection.

Plotkin continues, "In soulcentric romance, rather than attempting to make the other fit their preexisting fantasies, the lovers revel in endlessly exploring the mysterious nature of the Other in the here and now.... Our relationship will expose all the places we are emotionally blocked, blinded, wounded, caged, protected, or otherwise limited."[8]

We will experience fear, hurt, guilt, and anger, but from a place of maturity we will recognize these as opportunity for healing our personalities and moving on to soul-centered living.

Essence description

Oregon white truffle essence helps us to understand the complexities of the human psyche and the many masks used to cover insecurity and feelings of aloneness. It stands for concealed development. Oregon white truffle essence relates to imagination and grounding with nature. At first glance, these two terms appear diametrically opposed. But they are not. Truffle essence helps us rediscover the primal spark that adds feeling to life. It has an important role to play in discernment associated with the conceit, deceit, pretense, and hypocrisy widespread in society.

It has been found that women taking oral contraceptives are somehow exempt from accurate olfactory attraction. Oregon white truffle essence helps attune us to our primal instincts, irrespective of the timing of the menstrual cycle. Research has found that when women ovulate, they are attracted to men that are wild and dangerous. Oregon white truffle essence helps, on an emotional level, to discern the true motivation and recognize the sensual and exciting state associated with primal sex.

Women desire to raise their children with men who are similar to them in values and beliefs. The human gene pool may benefit from diversity and spark, but lasting love may be more possible in couples sharing common goals and dreams. Truffle mushroom essence may be useful for those individuals seeking a life partner. It appears the human leukocyte antigen plays a key role in what we call the spark of love. Two people meet and have an instant romantic attraction based on genetics. In no way does truffle mushroom essence block or prevent the pleasure associated with coupling, but it helps us discern the difference between lust and love.

PREPARATION: Oregon white truffle essence is produced by placing paper-thin slices into a small-scale distillation system and producing a hydrosol. This is combined one-to-one with brandy to produce the mother stock. The essence can be produced at any phase of the moon, but the new moon in any fire sign is ideal.

CASE STUDY: Rachael was twenty-eight years old and married for two years. She came to me due to menstrual problems associated with stopping the birth control pill. She had been put on the medication at age fourteen for painful, irregular periods, but now she wanted to have a child. The regularity of the menstrual cycle was resolved after two months with herbal therapy, using chasteberry (*Vitex agnus-castus*).

At our next meeting, she admitted the honeymoon phase of her relationship felt over, and she was not even sure she loved her husband. She remarked his body odor bothered her, even though he showered twice a day at her request. "I think I married my father," she said casually. I asked her to consider taking Oregon white truffle mushroom essence for a lunar cycle and keep a dream journal.

She returned the next month, looking sad and tearful. She noted in her journal that their love-making had become boring and infrequent. One written entry said, "All we had was great sex, and now even that is gone." I did not encourage her about making any decision. At her next visit three months later, she revealed they had separated, and her ex-husband was already in another relationship.

CORDYCEPS
(Cordyceps militaris)

INDICATIONS: addiction, allergies, transformation, altruism, euthanasia, rebirth, respiration

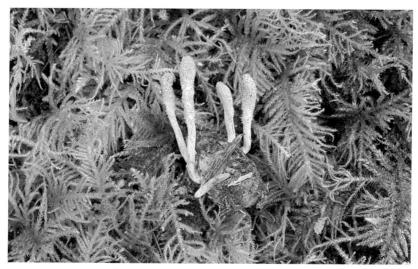

Cordyceps (*Cordyceps militaris* [L.] Link) (courtesy of Duane Sept)

Knowledge is a moth.
—CARLOS CASTANEDA

The atoms become like a moth, seeking out the region of higher laser intensity.
—STEVEN CHU

Everybody knows what a caterpillar is, and it doesn't look anything like a butterfly.
—LYNN MARGULIS

Metamorphosis by Franz Kafka is a worthy read for those individuals who believe in the common good and refuse to, or cannot, see the dark side of humanity. There may be a belief that biomedical progress and technology is an end that justifies the means. It helps us come to grips with life-and-death issues, including euthanasia, especially the lack of empowerment for patients facing end-of-life decisions.

A moth has three phases in life: the caterpillar, the pupa (cocoon), and the imago (the mature adult). It is not known how this takes place, but inside the caterpillar are cells called imaginal buds that contain the blueprint to allow it to imagine flying. Plotkin writes,

> *The caterpillar's immune system believes these imaginal cells are foreign and tries to destroy them, not unlike the way uninitiated human egos and their egocentric cultures often try to destroy the soul, nature, and the feminine.... It's as if the caterpillar doesn't realize its destiny is to become a butterfly. Likewise, the uninitiated ego doesn't recognize its destiny to become an agent for soul.[9]*

We die so that something new can be born.

Essence description

Cordyceps mushroom essence assists us on our soulful journey into the unknown. It provides a level of reassurance that, in the end, all the steps required are worth the sacrifice. It helps us get in touch with any denial around shadow exhibited by society in general. The mushroom essence may help us understand, or at least learn from, any recurring dreams of conspiracy or alien invaders. What are they telling us?

Cordyceps individuals may appear fragile or extremely sensitive to others, or they may feel judged by other people. Cordyceps mushroom essence may help assist opium and other narcotic withdrawal, combining well with earth star or liberty cap mushroom essences for this purpose.

There is an affinity for the lungs and the entire respiratory system. Ringing in the ears, dizziness, tinnitus, and Ménière's disease may all be helped. For the latter two conditions, Cordyceps mushroom essence combines well with wood ear.

Cordyceps essence is for people who are altruistic and sacrifice their own needs and wants for the greater good of society. Sacrificing ourselves is never a good strategy.

The mushroom essence may be helpful to those who react to, or reject, the impact of industry on their lives. On one level, this may manifest as allergies or sensitivity to environmental pollution, electromagnetic radiation, and so on. Individuals with sensitivities to food, chemicals, petroleum, medicines, and clothing may be helped by this mushroom essence. These highly sensitive people are the canary in the coal mine, awakening the consciousness of the general population to planetary pollution. Ironically, they may be dismissed as weak or inadequate, especially by those in denial of our environmental chaos. The mushroom essence helps bring awareness to these individuals and soothe any emotional backlash and judgment directed their way. At another level, it may relate to the anguish of modern life and its destruction of nature, community, and connectedness.

Another aspect of Cordyceps relates to generosity. When we are traveling our true path, the universe provides assistance, support, and encouragement from like-minded individuals. There is a reciprocal aspect that unites and aligns people with common goals and aspirations. Cordyceps essence brings awareness to this unfolding and promotes a "pay it forward" attitude.

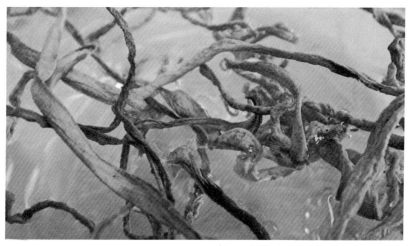

Cultivated *Cordyceps militaris* on rainwater

PREPARATION: Cordyceps essence is produced during the new moon in Scorpio. The fruiting bodies are placed on the surface of rainwater in a crystal bowl overnight. If need be, organic cultivated *C. militaris* may be substituted. Keep in mind that this mushroom has been handled by various people on its journey to your retail store; caution is advised for hypersensitive individuals.

CASE STUDY: Elaine was a fifteen-year-old student. Her mother brought her into my clinic for helps with allergies, dizziness, and difficulty breathing. She was experiencing recurring nightmares about alien abduction. She appeared pale, thin, and somewhat anorexic, but I was assured by her mother that she ate well. I examined her teeth for signs of bulimia and ruled it out. She had yet to experience the start of her menstrual cycles, but her mother assured me she was late herself when she was a young woman.

I first thought of artist's conk mushroom essence, as she had a fear of the outdoors, blaming her allergies on sensitivity to pollen from trees, grass, and flowers. I recognized the sensitivity of this individual and asked about her family history. Her grandmother on her mother's side was extremely ill with terminal bone cancer, suffering a great deal of pain. Elaine started to weep and acknowledged she was frightened. I recommended Cordyceps mushroom essence for a lunar cycle.

I received a call from her mother about two weeks later. Grandmother had passed on, and the daughter was present in her final moments. Her allergies and dizziness were gone, and she was gracefully moving through the phases of grieving. Her grandmother loved lilacs, and Elaine picked them from their yard for the funeral service, without reacting. One month later, her long delayed menarche began.

Lichens are unique life forms that are a symbiosis of algae and fungi. Some scientists use the term helotism *to describe a master-and-slave relationship. It is best, in my mind, to see the individual organisms for what they truly are, instead of using redundant reductionism.*

Lichen essences are prepared under solar influence due to their ability to photosynthesize and produce their own food.

WOLF LICHEN
(Letharia vulpina)

INDICATIONS: addiction, wisdom, solar plexus, anorexia, bulimia, self-confidence, gut feelings, charlatans, hypocrisy

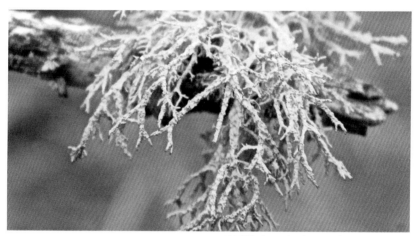

Wolf lichen (*Letharia vulpina* [L.] Hue)

From the lunar plexus I arose like a hungry trout and was caught fast on the sharp barbed hook that hangs inside all once-beautiful faces.
—LEONORA CARRINGTON

Wolf lichen (*Letharia vulpina*) is a bright yellow-green fluorescent color. As the name suggests, it is poisonous and was previously used to poison wild animals and to make arrow tips more effective in killing.

The concept of gorging and purging is a societal reflection of the North American lifestyle, with its indulgence in buying too many consumer goods and then selling them at garage sales in the following years. Could it be that bulimia is a metaphor for the splurge-and-purge consumerism that is rampant in society? It is a guttural response to our disconnection from soul. It represents the lack of nurturance presently found in modern-day society. Leonard Sax coined the term *anorexia of the soul,* first used in a 2007 *New York Times* article about the pressures on young girls.[1] This is associated with the drive to be perfect on the outside while feeling anxious, stressed, and frustrated on the inside.

Essence description

Wolf lichen essence helps to facilitate energy movement between the solar plexus and heart chakras. It soothes and strengthens the vagus nerve, associated with a plethora of issues around nurturing. It is a superb essence for the treatment of food addiction, anorexia nervosa, and cases of bulimia. The essence is not only for individuals dealing with these difficult issues but for the concerned extended family and health care workers helping those afflicted. Wolf lichen essence soothes both an overactive and underactive vagus nerve. In turn, there is influence on learning how to nurture ourselves.

The test point for this essence is at the base of the ribs. When there is stress, the area will be painful. Rubbing a few drops of essence into the area can be felt as a soothing and calming restoration. The solar plexus is one of the more significant nerve centers of the body, acting as a switchboard for digestive functions and gut-level instinct and reaction. It is the brain of the stomach, if you will, coordinating the secretion of saliva and the peristaltic action of the stomach, release of the gall bladder, and intestinal peristalsis. Instinctive wisdom, gut feelings, groundedness, and self-confidence are all affected.

An interesting book, *The Second Brain,* by Michael D. Gershon, explains in great detail the nervous system of our gut, or enteric nervous system. Various neurotransmitters, including serotonin and dopamine, are produce in this specialized intestinal tissue. Serotonin is widespread in nature and is produced and utilized by animals, fungi, and other plants for purposes of communication. Although well researched, the idea of a second brain in the stomach and intestine is not widely accepted nor recognized for its significance. It does explain the phrase "you are what you eat" in a convincing manner, however; or at least, we are what we digest and assimilate physically and emotionally. Or, what is eating you?

A wide range of problems is due to weakness of the solar plexus. Various nervous and muscular tensions arise, creating high blood pressure, migraines, and neuralgia throughout the body. All of our feelings arise from the solar plexus. When the solar plexus attempts to bypass the soul, difficulties arise. Negative thoughts such as jealousy, anger, prejudices, and possessiveness injure the solar plexus. Stomach problems stem from solar plexus crises.

Between the solar plexus and the heart is a place called the alcoholic ocean. It is here that many of today's addictive behaviors begin their journey. In a manner of speaking, the journey from the solar plexus to the heart is fraught with various intoxications.

The lunar plexus resides in the head, around the area of the sixth chakra. It is considered a cooling energy, as opposed to the fire in the solar. It is the center of calm reason and reflection, giving balance to the fire and emotion of the third charka.

Wolf lichen helps to facilitate a connection between the two plexuses, from the Latin *plectere,* meaning "to braid," "to twine," or "to fold." It is useful for detecting the wolf in sheep's clothing, the charlatans and hypocrites. It combines well with Oregon white truffle for help with this issue.

The common name, wolf lichen, is significant. Matthew Wood has contributed to our understanding of animal medicine, as defined by native North American healers:

> *As a representative of things medicinal, the wolf is most closely related to the animal instincts which reside in the solar plexus, the digestive tract to which it gives enervation, and the gallbladder, which is tied so closely to it by nerve reflexes. Wolves are known for their hunger. On a psychological level, wolf relates to the conscious*

ego, which dominates, organizes, rules, and sets boundaries. Yet, wolf also represents the ability to cross the boundaries, transform and move into something completely outside of known experience.[2]

This is the essence of twilight, and thin veils between the worlds. "The hour of the wolf is the time between night and dawn. It is the hour when most people die, when sleep is deepest, when nightmares are most palpable, when ghosts and demons hold sway. The hour of the wolf is also the hour when most children are born."[3]

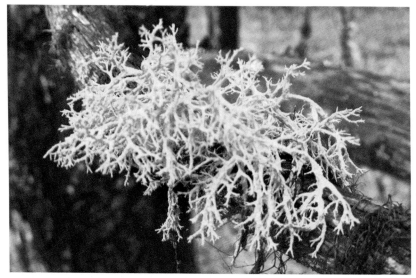

Wolf lichen

PREPARATION: Wolf lichen essence is produced in four hours of sunshine around the time of the full moon, in a crystal bowl with rainwater, preferably under the solar influence of Cancer. A few drops can be applied externally to the solar plexus when tender or sore.

CASE STUDY: Tania was a seventeen-year-old student. Her mother accompanied her daughter to my clinic, with concerns of anorexia, alternating with bouts of bulimia. She exhibited all the symptoms associated with this eating disorder. Her mother was a clinical psychologist. I noted a certain frigidity between them, making the interview difficult. The mother began answering questions directed toward Tania, so I asked if she could wait outside. She was very reluctant, but her daughter also insisted. The interview revealed the classic mother-daughter tension, with the added dimension of the psychologist-mother oversight. I suggested that the herb wood betony be taken internally for the solar plexus–brain connection, as well as a lunar cycle of wolf lichen essence, and that she keep a dream journal.

Four weeks later, Tania arrived at my office by herself, looking remarkably transformed. She appeared more self-confident and radiant. She asked me if the remedy was designed to allow her to see wolves. I replied, "Did you see wolves in your dreams?" She nodded and said not only in her dreams, but in real life. She was cross-country skiing with her friends two weeks earlier, and they saw seven of them roaming together at some distance. I asked her if she was familiar with the work of Clarissa Pinkola Estés, and her book *Women Who Run with the Wolves*. She replied no, but was interested. I asked about the anorexia-bulimia, and she said that after about ten days of the two remedies, she began to eat and enjoy food in a different way. She felt nourishment from her food, and began to shop for foods she really enjoyed. We talked about the importance of nurturing our body and our soul. She seemed to understand what I was saying.

Six months later, both mother and daughter came to thank me. They had both delved into the book I suggested, and through sharing its stories, started to rebuild their relationship. Tania daughter was considering taking psychology at university, which, not so secretly, pleased her mother a great deal.

REINDEER MOSS

(Cladonia rangiferina)

INDICATIONS: will, assertiveness, disassociation, fragmentation, jealousy, loss of self, scatteredness, feeling trapped

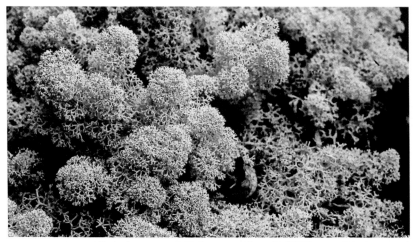

Reindeer moss (*Cladonia rangiferina* [L.] Weber ex F. H. Wiggers)

Resignation, not mystic, not detached, but resignation open-eyed, conscious, and informed by love, is the only one of our feelings for which it is impossible to become a sham.

—JOSEPH CONRAD

Reindeer moss is a long-lived lichen in northern climates. It is very sensitive to prolonged drought and can take up to one hundred years to recover after a fire. It is a major food source for caribou in the north.

Essence description

Reindeer moss essence is for those individuals who feel disassociated, fragmented, and scattered. There may be feelings of being trapped, used, or coerced by others. In some cases, they begin to take on the persona of those around them, leading to further alienation from their own self-identity. Individuals who may be helped with this essence may note they are easily swayed by the opinions of others. Tastes in music, film, food, and clothing will vary widely, depending on whom they are presently associated with. They may well be aware of this loss of identity, but there is little will or energy to assert themselves.

Associated with these feelings is an overwhelming tiredness, especially in the afternoon. Issues of jealousy may be present, even though there is no rational basis for the negative feeling. There may be suspicion of other people's motives. Consider combining or using yellow witch's butter or shaggy mane if the picture pattern fits. On a physical level, there may be blocked nostrils and sinuses, with sensation of cold. Or there may be a constant postnasal drip that has persisted for years.

What has led to such a state of inertia or resignation? The Platonic doctrine of anamnesis is the idea that we are born possessing all knowledge, and our soul once lived in reality but was trapped in our body. It once knew everything but forgot. Reindeer moss may help us "remember."

In many ways the state is reminiscent of the phrase "resistance is futile" from the science fiction series *Star Trek*. There is a certain resignation associated with this indifference; clients may say things like "Whatever" or "Who cares?" when asked about their lives. Reindeer moss essence is like a whiff of oxygen to the weak embers of will, helping rebuild a sense of hope and self-sufficiency.

Again, where did this state begin? Often this condition follows a serious illness, particularly of the nervous system, but may also be present due to emotional trauma in the first years of life. Plotkin suggests trauma at age two or three may result in the "loyal soldier" syndrome. These individuals will, throughout their lives, remain constantly vigilant to the early wound and react from this perspective.[4] Reindeer moss essence helps us to reconnect and nurture this young soul fragment toward integration.

Think back to events that excited you at a young age. This may be part of our soul path or soul purpose that has become buried under years of responsibility and duty. Feeling trapped today may have its roots in inappropriate comments from parents or teachers, giving rise to issues of self-esteem. In turn, striving to become the best we can is thwarted, leading to loss of self-identity, confusion, and resignation. If nothing is good enough, the psyche may translate this as "you" are not good enough.

Stuttering is one example of this state that may be helped by reindeer moss essence, combining well with luminescent Panellus mushroom essence, if the picture pattern fits.

PREPARATION: Reindeer moss essence is produced in a crystal bowl of rainwater in sunlight for four hours, during a new moon under Gemini or Virgo.

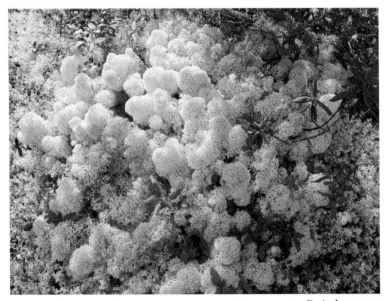

Reindeer moss

CASE STUDY: Keith was a twenty-four-year-old single pipefitter. He came into my office looking burdened and resigned. There was no life, no spark. He had suffered chronic sinusitis for over seven years. During our interview he would respond to my questions with "Whatever" or "Who cares?" as if he were talking to a parent or superior at work. I asked about him about his relationship with his father, and he mumbled something about him being a "hard ass." I asked him if they were in communication, and he shook his head. I suspected some trauma as a child but did not say anything further. I suggested a lunar cycle of reindeer moss essence, which perfectly fit his work schedule out of town.

He returned in four weeks, and there was a notable difference. He looks less disheveled and more present. I asked him if anything changed, and he replied, "Everything." Within a week of taking the drops, his father had phoned him, out of the blue, asking to borrow money. They had not spoken for seven years. They met at a bar, and it suddenly occurred to him that his father was an alcoholic. They had a fight, and Keith left without giving his father any money.

That night he had a dream, or a "memory," as he phrased it. He was seven years old and was helping his dad change a battery in their truck. It was too heavy for him and he dropped the new one, causing his father to shout, "You stupid ass." He awoke from the dream with his heart pounding and perspiration on his neck and brow. For the next four days, his nose secretions flowed nonstop. On the last day, a discharge of dark green frightened him, and he phoned me. I asked him to come in for a visit. I suggested that he had internalized and believed what his father said. I asked him what his father did for a living, and he said, "The same as me, a pipefitter." A lengthy discussion followed. I suggested he had been trying too hard to please his father. He was being responsible and dutiful at the expense of his own growth and enjoyment of life. He said nothing.

One month later, he sat in my office and let me know he had quit working as a pipefitter. He was going back to school to study geology, his real love. His chronic sinus problem was gone.

USNEA

(Dolichousnea longissima)

INDICATIONS: cravings, discontent, narcissism, work, occupation, tolerance, sunstroke

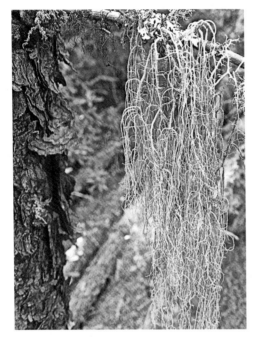

Usnea (*Dolichousnea longissima* [Acharius] Articus)

Before enlightenment, chop wood and haul water. After enlightenment, chop wood and haul water.

—CHINESE SAYING

When a condition or a problem becomes too great, humans have the protection of not thinking about it. But it goes inward and minces up with a lot of other things already there and what comes out is discontent and uneasiness, guilt and a compulsion to get something—anything—before it is all gone.

—JOHN STEINBECK

People should be sufficiently discontented to
feel there is something to live for.

—GEORGE BERNARD SHAW

Many people think of work as a function, forgetting its soul purpose. It is an ancient idea that we work on soul through our own everyday work. The alchemist calls this the opus, or "the work." Moore suggests:

> *We move closer to the soul's work when we go deeper than intellectual abstractions and imaginary fancies that do not well up from the more profound roots of feeling.... Work is an attempt to find an adequate alchemy that both wakens and satisfies the very root of being.... Work is fundamental to the opus because the whole point of life is the fabrication of soul.*[5]

Work is not the same as true vocation. It can be, but only if the inspiration for achievement is based on soul purpose.

Work is also not a means to an end. Money does not satisfy soul, but can buy a whole range of distractions. Moore continues:

> *Our work takes on narcissistic qualities when it does not serve well as a reflection of self. When that inherent reflection is lost, we become more concerned instead with how our work reflects on our reputations. We seek to repair our painful narcissism in the glow of achievement, and so we become distracted from the soul of the work for its sake. We are tempted to find satisfaction in the secondary rewards, such as money, prestige, and the trappings of success. It's obvious that climbing the ladder of success can easily lead to a loss of soul.*[6]

Essence description

Usnea lichen essence is useful for individuals in the helping or healing professions. At times, due to the desperate life-threatening situations and energies of the patients, there is danger of empathizing or identifying too strongly with patients and beginning to take on their "illness."

It is useful for those working in hospice and witnessing another journey of the soul.

Usnea essence helps retain boundaries, so that effective work can be carried out without endangering our own health and well-being. This can be subtle, but once observed, it can be recognized and easily dealt with.

Usnea essence is for restless discontent, those of us who are dissatisfied with life and tend to lack tolerance for others. We may be harmful to others, as well as ourselves. We may have a short temper and energetically burn the candle at both ends, leading to cravings that are harmful.

Sunstroke damage may have changed the personality, and this essence may bring back balance. One example of this is the use of food to stuff down emotions. An excellent book by Jack Schwarz, *It's Not What You Eat but What Eats You,* addresses the issue of body-mind connection with nutrition and vitality.

As might be expected, the lungs are most often affected. Traditionally, the lungs were associated with crying and the grieving process. Usnea essence helps protects those suffering from the *tuberculinum miasm,* recognized in homeopathic medicine. This makes sense when we consider the mycobacterial nature of this serious disease, and the treatment of patients with antibiotics and antifungal medications.

The miasmic taint or trait is more subtle and exists on a cellular or predisposed genetic level. It should be noted that usnea essence may temporarily increase skin irritations, particularly those with dry or weeping eczema. Caution is advised, and reducing the standard dosage by half will often help allay this acute bodily response.

PREPARATION: Usnea essence is produced under the influence of *both* sunshine and the full moon with rainwater in a crystal bowl for twenty-four hours under the solar influence of Gemini.

CASE STUDY: Hank was fifty-six years old, working as a furnace cleaning technician, and divorced for five years. The client was significantly overweight—well over three hundred pounds—with a choleric, red-faced, hypertensive profile. Diabesity was obvious, with high blood pressure, high blood sugar, and high cholesterol levels. He was

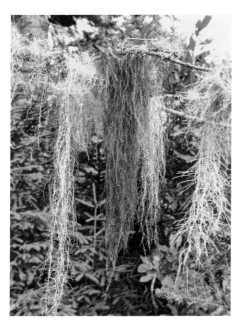

Usnea and other lichens

concerned with his lungs, and told me that when he was six years old he suffered from tuberculosis, contracted from an uncle. He smoked cigarettes and drank six to eight beers with his buddies after work. I was uncertain where to go, but I recommended dietary changes, some supplements for cardiovascular risks, and usnea mushroom essence at the last moment.

I was mildly surprised when he came back to see me about two months later. Something had changed, but I could not put my finger on it. He had lost twenty pounds, for which I congratulated him. I asked him if anything had occurred in the last eight weeks. He laughed. "I quit work," he said. About a month earlier, one of his drinking buddies had dropped dead at work of a heart attack. The shock was so profound that Hank could not go to work for a while, and when he did show up, he felt he could not be there. So he decided to retire.

We worked together on his health issues for the next eighteen months. He slimmed down to 210 pounds and stopped smoking and drinking beer. He joined Alcoholics Anonymous, where he met his new girlfriend.

SNAKE LIVERWORT

(Conocephalum conicum)

INDICATIONS: necrophilia, parasites, vampires, pregnancy, regeneration, transmutation, goth

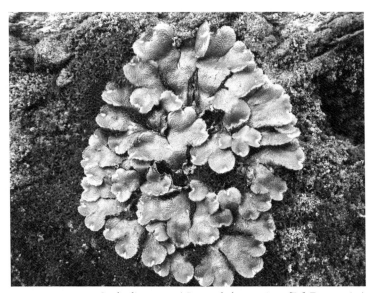

Snake liverwort (*Conocephalum conicum* [L.] Dumortier)

One perceives the fundamental essence of life in the living, not in the inanimate, in that which is changing, not in what is finished.
—GOETHE

Great scented liverwort, or snake liverwort, has a strong mushroom-like smell when crushed. It may be mixed with oils as an ointment for cuts and burns, and it inhibits the growth of microorganisms.

The Haida people call it *xud t'aangal,* or hair seal's tongue, while the southern Kwakiutl name is tongue on the ground. Other indigenous people such as the Ditidaht used it as an eye medicine. According to ethnobotanist Nancy J. Turner, various groups used snake liverwort for stoppage of urine.[1] One respondent mentioned this species was eaten by people having recurrent dreams of sex with the dead. If the treatment did not stop this night-time occurrence, it was believed that the dreamer would soon be joining their ancestors.

Fromm distinguished between a natural instinct of benign aggression, associated with protecting ourselves and survival, and malignant aggression, which is not physiological. Instead, it is a failure of character stemming from passion. It is existential and the need to make an impression on our world. One extreme of the destructive side is sadism; the other is the attraction to all that is dead. According to Fromm, necrophilia is both real and symbolic. The overall drive of the individual is a yearning for life to be over.[2] Dreams of dismembered parts or rooms full of skeletons can manifest. Dialogue with disowned parts of ourselves can help our soul journey.

The concept of soul as parasite is frightening to some individuals. Some traits include lifeless dry skin, compartmentalizing emotion and will, an interest in sickness, a tendency to wear dark colors or goth clothing, a dislike of anything bright, and a language filled with scatological words. Overall, there is a preference for the images of death over life.

Essence description

Snake liverwort essence is associated the concept of regeneration, cell division, and transmutation. In the case of regeneration, the essence may help promote increased production of cell growth and strengthen the ability to repair. On the other hand, it may help to slow down the excessive cell growth of cancer cells and skin cells related to psoriasis and similar conditions. For the latter, it combines well with velvet foot.

The essence is helpful to those who feel vulnerable to parasites. This could involve susceptibility to "energy vampires" in a social or workplace environment or in clinical practice, or individuals who believe their energy is waning due to perceived or real intestinal parasites. It combines well with lobster mushroom essence.

Another aspect that is helped by snake liverwort essence is the impression in pregnancy that the fetus is a parasite. Indeed, feeding from the mother can be interpreted as such when there is a lack of nurturance or resistance to the new experience. The essence, in this case, may help induce calm and acceptance in both mother and unborn child.

Early in utero experiences can influence the developing fetus. Bruce Lipton writes:

> *Now we know that the very same chemicals that shape a mother's experiences and behaviors cross the placenta and target the same cells and genes in the fetus that they do in the mother. The consequence is that the developing fetus, bathed in the same blood chemistry as the mother, experiences the same emotions and physiology as the mother. The fetus, for example, absorbs cortisol and other stress hormones if the mother is chronically anxious. If the child is unwanted for any reason, the fetus is bathed in the chemicals of rejection.*[3]

Snake liverwort essence may reinforce the ability of the body to transmute one element into another. Organic silica, for example, is utilized by the body for the formation of calcium. Organic manganese may be transmuted into organic iron, and so on. For this purpose, add two drops of snake liverwort essence to your herbal preparation at the last minute before ingestion. For more information, refer to the fascinating work of C. Louis Kervran in *Biological Transmutations*.[4]

Snake liverwort is associated with the moon in Scorpio and the planet Pluto.

PREPARATION: Ideally, this essence is produced under sunlight under the influence of either the moon in Scorpio or the planet Pluto. The liverwort is placed on rainwater in a crystal bowl for four hours. Bryophytes are plants.

CASE STUDY: Tracy was twenty-nine years old, single, and working as a bartender. She came into my office wearing a black T-shirt with picture of a vampire and the words "Bloody Hell." She had very pale, dry skin and used words alluding to human feces in her colorful language. She was tattooed over most of her exposed body parts, with snakes being a common theme.

I learned Tracy had a boyfriend, and she alluded to their mutual enjoyment of sadomasochistic sex. She had recently found out she was pregnant and wanted advice about achieving a miscarriage with herbs. I told her this was not something I could help her with, and she rose to leave. She repeated "shit, shit, shit," three times under her breath as she prepared to exit. I asked if she really wanted to end the pregnancy, or if she was frightened and uncertain if she could go full term and be a good mother. She turned, and tears began to fall. She sat down and told me the baby felt like a parasite, that it was feeding off of her. I assured her that it was dependent on her for food, but that is was definitely not a parasite, but a developing human being. I offered to help her with nutritional advice and said snake liverwort essence may help her deal with these feelings of parasitism.

I suggested she keep a dream journal. We met in my office one lunar cycle later. She looked different. She had moved out of her boyfriend's apartment and into a house with three other women. I asked about any dreams and her journal. She admitted to not doing the "homework," but shared one dream she had had the other night. She was floating at night in a warm ocean, feeling content, when a tidal wave picked her up and smashed her down on the beach. She felt bruised, bleeding, and in pain. And then she woke up. I asked about her relationship with her own mother and her birthing experience. She had been adopted at an early age, and did not know her birth mother. She started to cry. "Please help keep my baby and me healthy," she said. And seven months later, she gave birth to a beautiful seven pound baby boy with a head full of dark, black hair.

KEY ISSUES AND CONDITIONS

abandonment	shiitake
abuse	fly agaric
acceptance	oyster
addiction	liberty cap, earth star, Cordyceps, Agaricus, wolf lichen, turkey tail
adoption	shiitake
aggression	tinder conk, giant puffball
agitation	cinnabar
alchemy	chicken of the woods
Alcoholics Anonymous	earth star
alienation	Agaricus
aliens	cinnabar
allergies	Cordyceps
aloneness	algae maze, iqmik
aloofness	oyster
altruism	Cordyceps, dog stinkhorn
Alzheimer's disease	comb tooth
anal issues	giant puffball
andropause	chicken of the woods
anger	cinnabar, tinder conk, fly agaric
animation	chicken of the woods
anorexia	wolf lichen
antibiotics	shiitake
anxiety	birch polypore, giant puffball
appreciation (lack of)	birch polypore
arrogance	oyster, algae maze
arthritis	red-belted conk, fly agaric
assertiveness	reindeer moss

atherosclerosis	red-belted conk
attention	Agaricus, oyster
attention deficit hyperactivity disorder/space	algae maze
auditory issues	wood ear
authenticity	turkey tail, varnish conk, morel
authority figures	liberty cap, fly agaric
autism spectrum disorder	wood ear
awareness	Agaricus, oyster
belief	chaga, red-belted conk, Grifola
biomedicine	Grifola, Agaricus
birth	fairy ring
black sheep	maze gill
bladder	giant puffball
body language	luminescent Panellus
body parts	green death cap
boredom	badia, Oregon white truffle
boundaries	oyster, usnea
bulimia	wolf lichen
burning	oyster
butterfly	badia, Cordyceps
cancer	chaga, green death cap
catalyst	wrinkled peach
cellular memory	comb tooth
chaos	Peziza
charlatan	Oregon white truffle, wolf lichen
chastity	rosy conk
chronic fatigue syndrome	split gill
circadian rhythm	split gill, chaga, fairy ring
circumcision	dog stinkhorn
cleanliness	Peziza
clear thinking	green elf cup
coercion	reindeer moss

communication	green elf cup, luminescent Panellus, wood ear
compassion	green elf cup
competition	giant puffball
compulsion	dog's stinkhorn
conceit	oyster
concentration	comb tooth
conditional love	iqmik
conformity	varnish conk
congestion	rosy conk
constriction	chaga, rosy conk, algae maze
consumerism	liberty cap
contraction	fly agaric
contrariness	diamond willow
control	Peziza, shiitake, shaggy mane, dog stinkhorn
corporate	dog stinkhorn
cosmic connection	earth star
courage	diamond willow
cravings	usnea
creativity	fly agaric
crises of identity	maze gill
criticism	fly agaric, blue Albatrellus, turkey tail, iqmik
crone	badia, honey
crying	red-belted conk, artist's conk, diamond willow
cultural awareness	shiitake
dancing	liberty cap, fairy ring
death	varnish conk, iqmik, snake liverwort, Cordyceps
deceit	oyster
deception	red-belted conk
defensiveness	green death cap

delusions	lobster
denial	red-belted conk, liberty cap
depression	green death cap, cinnabar, birch polypore, fly agaric
despair	artist's conk
destruction	giant puffball, algae maze
detachment	Peziza
diamonds	green death cap
disassociation	reindeer moss
discernment	red-belted conk, Oregon white truffle
discomfort	velvet foot
discontent	usnea, velvet foot
discrimination	shiitake
dis-ease	Grifola
disintegration	iqmik
distinctness	chicken of the woods
divinity	diamond willow
divorce	oyster
DMT	chaga
DNA	morel
dog	green death cap
doors of perception	wood ear
dopamine	wolf lichen
dreams	green death cap, bird's nest, iqmik, Cordyceps, agarikon, snake liverwort, cinnabar, oyster, yellow witch's butter, chicken of the woods
drowning	oyster
Dupuytren's contracture	fly agaric
earthquakes	green death cap
eczema	velvet foot, usnea
egotism	oyster, yellow witch's butter
elder wisdom	honey
emotional flexibility	badia

empathy	artist's conk, dog stinkhorn, usnea
empty nest syndrome	badia
enlightenment	rosy conk
entitlement	cinnabar
envy	yellow witch's butter, birch polypore, turkey tail
equality	Oregon white truffle
erotic parts	giant puffball
escapism	morel
euthanasia	Cordyceps
evidence based medicine	hen of the woods
exhaustion	lobster
expansion and contraction	green death cap
exposure	velvet foot
extroversion	earth star, morel
faith	agarikon
family	green death cap
fasting	iqmik, diamond willow
fear	tinder conk, snake liverwort, shiitake, morel, liberty cap
fear of success	iqmik
fear of water	agarikon
feeling/thinking from the heart	green elf cup, green death cap
femininity	blue Albatrellus, artist's conk, tinder conk
fertility	fairy ring
flexibility	red-belted conk, Agaricus, yellow witch's butter, badia, honey
floods	agarikon
fool, the	diamond willow
foreboding	cinnabar
fragmentation	reindeer moss, Peziza
freedom	wrinkled peach, morel, Oregon white truffle

friendship	honey, green elf cup
frustration	cinnabar, badia, shaggy mane, giant puffball
future	cinnabar
gallbladder	cinnabar, honey, wolf lichen
gender identity	dog stinkhorn
genital issues	giant puffball
gloominess	blue Albatrellus
grace	birch polypore
gratefulness	oyster
gregariousness	chicken of the woods
groundedness	Oregon white truffle
guilt	split gill, cinnabar
gut feelings	wolf lichen
hallucinations	wood ear
harmony	Grifola
health	Grifola
heart	tinder conk, green elf cup
hero's journey	dog stinkhorn
humility	oyster
hyperactivity	Agaricus
hypocrisy	Oregon white truffle
identity	maze gill, reindeer moss
imagination	fly agaric, Oregon white truffle
imbalance	chicken of the woods
immortality	varnish conk
impatience	cinnabar, earth star
impulsiveness	earth star
indoctrination	chaga, green death cap
inertia	birch polypore
inflammation	rosy conk
inflexibility	fly agaric
inner child	fairy ring

inner voice	wood ear
insecurity	Oregon white truffle, fly agaric
insomnia	split gill
inspiration	chicken of the woods
integrative health	Grifola
intimacy	morel
introversion	luminescent Panellus, chicken of the woods, blue Albatrellus, morel
invisibility	lobster
isolation	algae maze
jealousy	yellow witch's butter, reindeer moss, shaggy mane
Jekyll & Hyde	earth star
judgment	shiitake, tinder conk, green elf cup, Grifola
karma	chaga
labor	fairy ring
lamenting	diamond willow
law	elf cup
liberty	liberty cap, Oregon white truffle
life and death	Cordyceps
listening	wood ear
loneliness	algae maze, iqmik
loss of a loved one	earth star
loss of purpose	badia
loss of self	reindeer moss
love	Peziza, Oregon white Truffle
loyal soldier syndrome	reindeer moss
lucid dreaming	bird's nest
lunar plexus	wolf lichen
lungs	usnea
lust	rosy conk, Oregon white truffle
manhood	dog stinkhorn
martyrdom	cinnabar, blue Albatrellus

masculinity	shaggy mane, artist's conk, tinder conk, dog stinkhorn
mask	morel
masturbation	giant puffball
materialism	earth star, velvet foot
melancholy	birch polypore
melatonin	chaga, split gill, fairy ring
memory	comb tooth
Ménière's disease	wood ear, Cordyceps
menopause	chicken of the woods
menstruation	fairy ring
mental illness	wood ear
midlife crisis	honey, badia
misery	yellow witch's butter
money	dog's stinkhorn, varnish conk, usnea
monotony	badia
mooning	giant puffball
music	Grifola
nakedness	velvet foot
narcissism	usnea
nature deficit disorder	Agaricus, artist's conk
nature versus nurture	artist's conk
necrophilia	snake liverwort
nervous tension	maze gill
neuroses	Peziza, algae maze
nonverbal	luminescent Panellus
numbness	fly agaric
obsession	badia, dog stinkhorn, giant puffball, turkey tail
obsessive-compulsive	giant puffball, algae maze
occult	lobster
occupation/profession	shaggy mane, usnea
optimism	blue Albatrellus, morel, earth star

oral fixation	giant puffball
overwhelmed feeling	blue Albatrellus
pain	rosy conk, iqmik, fly agaric
pancreas	cinnabar
Paranoia	Peziza, yellow witch's butter
parasites	snake liverwort
Parkinson's disease	fly agaric
passion	chicken of the woods
past	comb tooth
perfection	Peziza, giant puffball
pessimism	blue Albatrellus, morel
pineal gland	chaga, split gill
pioneer spirit	birch polypore
pissed off	giant puffball
pituitary	chaga, red-belted conk
pleasure	Grifola
pornography	shaggy mane, giant puffball
post–traumatic stress	varnish conk
power	diamond willow
pregnancy	snake liverwort, fairy ring
premature birth	lobster
premonition	lobster
pride	oyster
primal spark	Oregon white truffle
professional sports	shaggy mane
projection	honey, bird's nest, morel, oyster
projective identification	morel
protection	diamond willow
psoriasis	velvet foot, snake liverwort
psychoses	algae maze
psychosomatic illness	badia
purpose (loss of)	badia
pursuit	green death cap

racism	shiitake
rebirth	Cordyceps, agarikon
receptiveness	giant puffball
regeneration	snake liverwort
rejection	green death cap, fly agaric
relationship	wrinkled peach
relaxation	turkey tail, lobster, diamond willow
religion	chaga, fly agaric, rosy conk, green death cap
repetition	green death cap
repression	rosy conk, green death cap
resentment	fly agaric
resistance	wrinkled peach
respiration	Cordyceps, usnea
responsibility	red-belted conk, velvet foot
reverse warrior	diamond willow
rigidity	red-belted conk
Ritalin	Agaricus
romantic feelings	blue Albatrellus, Oregon white truffle
sadism	snake liverwort
sadness	birch polypore
Saturn	birch polypore, Oregon white truffle
scatteredness	reindeer moss
schizophrenia	wood ear
scleroderma	fly agaric
second brain	wolf lichen
secrecy	morel
self-arousal	giant puffball
self-awareness	death cap, luminescent Panellus
self-confidence	wolf lichen
self-criticism	iqmik
self-deprecation	iqmik, oyster
self-destruction	iqmik

self-doubt	chaga
self-fulfilling prophecy	lobster, blue Albatrellus
self-identity	maze gill
self-image	luminescent Panellus
self-love	varnish conk, wrinkled peach
self-pity	badia
sensory gating	wood ear
serotonin	wolf lichen
sexism	shaggy mane
sexual abuse	fly agaric, giant puffball, split gill
sexuality	rosy conk, split gill, Oregon white truffle
shadow work	shiitake, morel, Oregon white truffle, oyster, diamond willow
shouting	cinnabar
silence	wood ear
sin	split gill, giant puffball, yellow witch's butter, Oregon white truffle
skin	velvet foot, cinnabar, snake liverwort, giant puffball
solar plexus	wolf lichen, maze gill
sorrow	green death cap
soul	usnea, yellow witch's butter, Grifola, diamond willow
spirituality	agarikon, rosy conk
stage fright	luminescent Panellus
stagnation	badia
stress	Agaricus
stillness	wood ear
stuttering	luminescent Panellus, reindeer moss
subconscious	luminescent Panellus
sulfur	chicken of the woods
sunstroke	usnea
survival instincts	Agaricus
tantric sex	rosy conk

tears	red-belted conk
television	elf cup, earth star, turkey tail
temper	cinnabar, usnea
tension	hen of the woods
time	varnish conk, cinnabar
tinnitus	wood ear, Cordyceps
tolerance	usnea
traditional roles	shaggy mane
transformation	varnish conk, Cordyceps
transmutation	snake liverwort
transparency	diamond willow
trapped feeling	reindeer moss, chicken of the woods
travel	shiitake
true path	varnish conk, turkey tail, diamond willow
trust	iqmik
unconditionality	wrinkled peach
ungroundedness	Peziza
urban-rural disconnect	Agaricus
urethra fixation	giant puffball
uro-genital issues	rosy conk
vagus nerve	wolf lichen
vampires	snake liverwort, lobster
verbal communication	wood ear
veterinary issues	Agaricus
victim	cinnabar
vision quest	iqmik, diamond willow
voice-hearing	wood ear
vulnerability	lobster
water	agarikon
well-being	wrinkled peach, Grifola, usnea
will	green death cap, reindeer moss
wisdom	wolf lichen, badia, chicken of the woods, yellow witch's butter

womb	dog stinkhorn, algae maze
writer's block	shaggy mane, elf cup, luminescent Panellus
zest	Agaricus
zombies	lobster

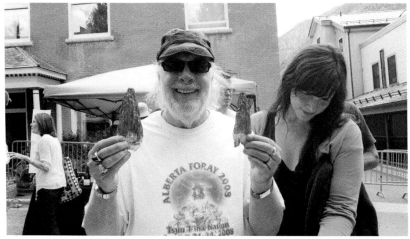

The author enjoying a morel dilemma

APPENDIX A:
PLANETARY MUSHROOM
CORRESPONDENCES

This chart is a list of planetary mushroom correspondences based on the doctrine of signatures. Each planet emits an energy expressed as an archetypal force that gives rise to the morphology and spiritual properties of physical manifestations, and in this chart, mushrooms. In alchemical philosophy, upon death, everything returns to its Sephiroth (Tree of Life), which correlates to planetary energy. This is the energy that emits and projects them onto the terrestrial plane. Each planet carries particular energetics and correspondence to organs and body systems.

Planet	Day	Main Organ	2nd Organ	System	Tissue	Action	Mushroom	Secondary Rulers
Sun	Sunday	Heart	Blood	Circulatory	Plasma	Hot/Dry	Cantharellus formosus (Chanterelle)	Mercury/Saturn
							Boletus edulis (King Bolete)	Mercury
							Ganoderma lucidum (Reishi)	Mercury
							Ganoderma oregonense (Oregon Reishi)	Mercury
							Laetiporus s.ulphureus (Chicken of the Woods)	Mars
Moon	Monday	Brain	Stomach	Nervous	Marrow	Cold/Moist	Coprinus comatus (Shaggy Mane)	Mars/Mercury
							Hericium erinaceus (Lion's Mane)	Mercury/Saturn
							Schizophyllum commune (Split Gill Polypore)	Mercury
							Pseudohydnum gelatinosum (Jelly Tooth)	Sun
							Tremella mesenterica (Witch's Butter)	Mercury
Mars	Tuesday	Blood	Gallbladder	Immune	Muscles/Tendons	Hot/Dry	Cordyceps spp.	Sun
							Fomitopsis pinicola (Red Belted Polypore)	Sun
							Inonotus obliquus (Chaga)	Jupiter/Venus
							Piptoporus betulinus (Birch Polypore)	Jupiter/Saturn
							Russula integra	Sun
Mercury	Wednesday	Lungs	Mind	Respiratory	Lymph	Cold/Dry	Grifola frondcsa (Maitake)	Jupiter/Saturn
							Pleurotus ostreatus (Oyster)	Moon
							Psilocybe cubensis	Saturn
							Stropharia rugosoannulata (King Stropharia)	Saturn
Jupiter	Thursday	Liver	Gallbladder	Metabolic	Fat	Warm/Moist	Agaricus bisporus (Portobello)	Saturn
							Fomitopsis officinalis (Agarikon)	Saturn
							Lentinula edoces (Shiitake)	Saturn
Venus	Friday	Kidney	Bladder	Genitourinary	Mucous	Warm/Dry	Amanita muscaria (Fly Agaric)	Jupiter
							Flammulina velutipes (Enoki)	Moon
							Ganoderma applanatum (Artist Conk)	Mercury/Saturn
							Trametes versicolor (Turkey Tail)	Jupiter/Saturn
Saturn	Saturday	Spleen	Bone/Joint	Skeletal/Structural	Bones	Cold/Dry	Claviceps purpurea (Rye Ergot)	Mercury
							Fomes fomentarius (Tinder Conk)	Venus
							Phellinus igniarius (Shelf Fungus)	Moon/Jupiter

Credit: Appendix A is adapted from a chart by Jason Scott and Peter McCoy, from *Radical Mycology* by Peter McCoy.

NOTES

Foreword

1. Edward Bach, *Heal Thyself: An Explanation of the Real Cause and Cure of Disease* (London: C. W. Daniel, 1931), 6.

Introduction

1. "Metaphor of Mushrooms," Sri Lanka *Sunday Times* 41:24, November 12, 2006.
2. Tomas Zilvar and Radeq Brousil, "The Mushroom Whisperer," *Vice,* October 27, 2011, www.vice.com/read/Vaclav-Halek-makes-mushroom -music.
3. David Richo, *How to Be an Adult: A Handbook on Psychological and Spiritual Integration* (New York: Paulist Press, 2002), ix, 3–5.
4. Martin W. Ball, *Mushroom Wisdom: How Shamans Cultivate Spiritual Consciousness* (Oakland, CA: Ronin, 2006), 49–50.
5. Clare G. Harvey, Andreas Korte, George Lewith, and Richard Gerber, *The Practitioner's Encyclopedia of Flower Remedies: The Definitive Guide to All Flower Essences, Their Making and Uses* (Philadelphia: Singing Dragon, 2015), 153.

The Journey of Discovering Mushroom Essences

1. Julia Graves, *The Language of Plants: A Guide to the Doctrine of Signatures* (Great Barrington, MA: Lindisfarne, 2012), 33.
2. Matthew Wood, *The Book of Herbal Wisdom: Using Plants as Medicine* (Berkeley, CA: North Atlantic Books, 1997), 23.

The Fungal-Chemical Process

1. C. G. Jung, "The Aims of Psychotherapy," *The Collected Works of C. G. Jung, Vol. 16: The Practice of Psychotherapy* (New York: Pantheon, 1953), 115–16.

How to Prepare and Use Mushroom Essences

1. Anne Baring, and Jules Cashford, *The Myth of the Goddess: Evolution of an Image* (New York: Viking Arkana, 1991), 20.
2. Ibid., 21.

Polypores (Polyporaceae)

1. Frans Vermeulen, *Fungi: Kingdom Fungi* (Haarlem, Netherlands: Emryss, 2007), 188.
2. George F. Will, "Handbook Suggests That Deviations from 'Normality' Are Disorders," *Washington Post,* February 28, 2010.
3. Richard Louv, "Children and Nature Movement: How a Movement Is Forming and How You Can Get Involved," March 2008, http:// richardlouv.com/books/last-child/children-nature-movement/.
4. Ralph Twentyman, *The Science and Art of Healing* (Edinburgh: Floris Books, 1989), 242–43.
5. Jung, "Aims of Psychotherapy," 98.
6. Brian G. Dias and Kerry J. Ressler, "Parental Olfactory Experience Influences Behavior and Neural Structure in Subsequent Generations," *Nature Neuroscience* 17 (2014), 89–96, doi:10.1038/nn.3594.
7. Sam Keen, *Fire in the Belly: On Being a Man* (New York: Bantam, 1991), 41–42.
8. Susanne S. Pedersen, Pedro A. Lemos, Priya R. van Vooren, Tommy K. K. Liu, Joost Daemen, Ruud A. M. Erdman, Pieter C. Smits, et al., "Type D Personality Predicts Death or Myocardial Infarction after Bare Metal Stent or Sirolimus-Eluting Stent Implantation," *Journal of the American College of Cardiology* 44 (5:2004), 997–1001, doi:10.1016/j.jacc.2004.05.064.
9. Jean Decety, Jason M. Cowell, Kang Lee, Randa Mahasneh, Susan Malcolm-Smith, Bilge Selcuk, and Xinyue Zhou, "The Negative Association between Religiousness and Children's Altruism across the World," *Current Biology* 25:22 (November 16, 2015), 2951–55, doi:10.1016/j.cub.2015.09.056.
10. Jack Schwarz, *It's Not What You Eat but What Eats You* (Berkeley, CA: Celestial Arts, 1988), 103–4.
11. Thomas Moore, *Care of the Soul: A Guide for Cultivating Depth and Sacredness in Everyday Life* (New York: Harper Collins, 1992), 169.
12. Schwarz, *It's Not What You Eat,* 104.
13. Matthew Wood, *Vitalism: The History of Herbalism, Homeopathy, and Flower Essences* (Berkeley, CA: North Atlantic, 2000), 29–30.
14. Twentyman, *Science and Art of Healing,* 90.

15. Joseph Campbell, *The Hero with a Thousand Faces* (New York: Pantheon, 1949), 211.

16. Moore, *Care of the Soul,* 136.

17. Ibid., 138.

18. Ibid., 139.

19. Bill Plotkin, *Soulcraft: Crossing into the Mysteries of Nature and Psyche* (Novato, CA: New World Library, 2003), 288.

20. Johnthomas Didymus, "Religious Fundamentalism Could Soon Be Treated as Mental Illness," Digital Journal, June 2, 2013, http://www. digitaljournal.com/article/351347.

21. José Stevens, *Transforming Your Dragons: Turning Personality Fear Patterns into Personal Power* (Santa Fe, NM: Bear and Co., 1994), 112.

22. R. C. Peck, "Psychological Developments in the Second Half of Life," in *Middle Age and Aging: A Reader in Social Psychology,* ed. Bernice L. Neugarten (Chicago: University of Chicago Press, 1968), 88–92.

23. C. G. Jung, *Archetypes and the Collective Unconscious,* trans. R. F. C. Hull (Princeton, NJ: Princeton University Press, 1959), 21–22.

24. Plotkin, *Soulcraft,* 134.

25. Sarah Dessen and Nancy Brennan, *Lock and Key: A Novel* (New York: Viking, 2008), quoting Mary Martha Sherwood, *The Monk of Cimiés,* 1834.

26. Sumathi Reddy, "A Perfect Dose of Pessimism," *Wall Street Journal,* August 5, 2014, quoting Frieder R. Lang, David Weiss, Denis Gerstorf, and Gert G. Wagner, "Forecasting Life Satisfaction across Adulthood: Benefits of Seeing a Dark Future?" *Psychology and Aging* 28 (1: March 2013), 249–61, doi:10.1037/a0030797.

27. Reddy, "Perfect Dose," quoting Suzanne C. Segerstrom, *Breaking Murphy's Law: How Optimists Get What They Want from Life—and Pessimists Can Too* (New York: Guilford Press, 2006).

28. Reddy, "Perfect Dose," quoting Katherine J. Bangen, Marianne Bergheim, Allison R. Kaup, Heline Mirzakhanian, Christina E. Wierenga, Dilip V. Jeste, and Lisa T. Eyler, "Brains of Optimistic Older Adults Respond Less to Fearful Faces," *Journal of Neuropsychiatry and Clinical Neurosciences* 26 (2: spring 2014), 155–63, doi:10.1176/appi.neuropsych.12090231.

29. Reddy, "Perfect Dose," quoting Erin M. O'Mara, James K. McNulty, and B. R. Karney, "Positively Biased Appraisals in Everyday Life: When Do They Benefit Mental Health and When Do They Harm It?" *Journal of Personality and Social Psychology* 101 (3: September 2011), 415–32, doi:10.1037/a0023332.

30. Elizabeth Kolbert, "Thomas Friedman: Hope for a Hot, Flat and Crowded World," *Yale Environment 360,* October 9, 2008.

31. C. G. Jung, *Memories, Dreams, Reflections* (New York: Pantheon, 1963), 356.

32. Plotkin, *Soulcraft,* 282.

33. Moore, *Care of the Soul,* 260.

34. Ibid.

35. Sándor Ferenczi, Judith Dupont, Michael Balint, and Nicola Zarday Jackson, *The Clinical Diary of Sándor Ferenczi* (Cambridge, MA: Harvard University Press, 1995), 5.

36. Bach, *Heal Thyself,* 2.

37. Moore, *Care of the Soul,* 162.

Gilled Mushrooms (Basidiomycetes)

1. Graves, *Language of Plants,* 70.

2. Edward C. Whitmont, *The Symbolic Quest: Basic Concepts of Analytical Psychology* (Princeton, NJ: Princeton University Press, 1969), 63.

3. C. G. Jung, *The Undiscovered Self* (New York: Little, Brown, 1958), 73.

4. Joachim-Ernst Berendt, *The Third Ear: On Listening to the World,* trans. Tim Nevill (Shaftesbury, UK: Element, 1988), 177.

5. Moore, *Care of the Soul,* 163.

6. Michael Barreto, "Astrology Affects the Yield of Shiitake Mushrooms," Aztro1.com, May 28, 2014, www.aztro1.com/research/biodynamic -mushroom-farming.htm.

7. Whitmont, *Symbolic Quest,* 142.

8. Twentyman, *Science and Art of Healing,* 223–24.

9. C. G. Jung, *Dream Analysis: Notes of the Seminar Given in 1928–1930* (London: Routledge & Kegan Paul, 1984).

10. Whitmont, *Symbolic Quest,* 165.

11. Ibid.

12. Bach, *Heal Thyself,* 12.

13. G. I. Gurdjieff, *Meetings with Remarkable Men,* trans. A. R. Orage (New York: E. P. Dutton, 1963), 36.

14. Eric Dubay, personal communication with the author.

15. Ball, *Mushroom Wisdom,* 50.

16. Plotkin, *Soulcraft,* 90.

17. James A. Coan, Hillary S. Schaefer, and Richard J. Davidson, "Lending a Hand: Social Regulation of the Neural Response to Threat," *Psychological Science* 17:12 (December 2006), 1032–39, doi:10.1111/j.1467-9280.2006.01832.x.

18. Sarah L. Master, Naomi I. Eisenberger, Shelley E. Taylor, Bruce D. Naliboff, David Shirinyan, and Matthew D. Lieberman, "A Picture's Worth:

Partner Photographs Reduce Experimentally Induced Pain," *Psychological Science* 20:11 (November 2009), 1316–18, doi:10.1111/j.1467-9280.2009.02444.x.

19. Clark Heinrich, *Magic Mushrooms in Religion and Alchemy* (Rochester, VT: Park Street Press, 2002); John A. Rush, *The Mushroom in Christian Art: The Identity of Jesus in the Development of Christianity* (Berkeley, CA: North Atlantic Books, 2011); J. R. Irvin and Jack Herer, *The Holy Mushroom: Evidence of Mushrooms in Judeo-Christianity* (Gnostic Media Research & Pub., 2008).

20. M. Zimecki, "The Lunar Cycle: Effects on Human and Animal Behavior and Physiology," *Poste py higieny i medycyny dos wiadczalnej* (Warsaw) 60 (2006): 1–7.

21. Nor Hall, *The Moon and the Virgin: Reflections on the Archetypal Feminine* (New York: Harper & Row, 1980), 4.

22. Ibid.

23. Richard Louv, *Last Child in the Woods: Saving Our Children from Nature-Deficit Disorder* (Chapel Hill, NC: Algonquin Books, 2006), 36.

24. Plotkin, *Soulcraft,* 89.

25. Berendt, *Third Ear,* 168.

26. Plotkin, *Soulcraft,* 280–81.

27. Ibid., 280–81.

28. Robert Bly, *A Little Book on the Human Shadow* (New York: HarperCollins, 1988), 15.

Gasteromycetes

1. Lance M. Dodes and Zachary Dodes, *The Sober Truth: Debunking the Bad Science Behind 12-Step Programs and the Rehab Industry* (Boston: Beacon Press, 2014), 1.

2. Keen, *Fire in the Belly,* 14–15.

3. Ibid., 78–79.

4. Moore, *Care of the Soul,* 190.

5. Elisa Filevich, Martin Dresler, Timothy R. Brick, and Simone Kühn, "Metacognitive Mechanisms Underlying Lucid Dreaming," *The Journal of Neuroscience* 35 (3: January 21, 2015), 1082–88, doi:10.1523/JNEUROSCI.3342-14.2015.

6. Whitmont, *Symbolic Quest,* 240.

7. Ibid., 243.

8. Ibid., 244.

Tremellales

1. Moore, *Care of the Soul,* 96.
2. Ibid., 101.
3. George Orwell, "In Front of Your Nose: 1945–1950," in George Orwell, Sonia Orwell, and Ian Angus, *The Collected Essays, Journalism, and Letters of George Orwell* (New York: Harcourt, Brace, 1968).
4. Ibid., 102.
5. Ibid, 114.
6. Herodotus, *The Histories,* 1.8.
7. William Blake, *The Marriage of Heaven and Hell,* 17932 object 14.
8. Stephen Harrod Buhner, *Plant Intelligence and the Imaginal Realm: Beyond the Doors of Perception into the Dreaming Earth* (Rochester, VT: Bear & Co., 2014), 19.
9. Berendt, *Third Ear,* 129.

Ascomycetes

1. K. M. Abenheimer, "The Ego as Subject," in *The Reality of the Psyche,* ed. Joseph B. Wheelwright (New York: Putnam, 1968), 61–73.
2. Buhner, *Plant Intelligence,* 508.
3. Albert Einstein, *Cosmic Religion: With Other Opinions and Aphorisms* (New York: Covici-Friede, 1931), 97.
4. Lazaris, "Working with Your Shadow I: An Imperative on the Spiritual Path," *New Moon Rising* 42 (March–April 1996), http://www.nmrjournal .com/zine/archive/issues/42/444.htm.
5. Plotkin, *Soulcraft,* 274, quoting James Hillman, *Re-Visioning Psychology* (New York: Harper & Row, 1975).
6. Plotkin, *Soulcraft,* 274.
7. Ibid., 280.
8. Ibid., 285.
9. Ibid., 78.

Lichens

1. Sara Rimer, "For Girls, It's Be Yourself, and Be Perfect, Too," *New York Times,* April 1, 2007.
2. Wood, *Book of Herbal Wisdom,* 13.
3. Hall, *Moon and the Virgin,* 117.
4. Plotkin, *Soulcraft,* 91–96.

5. Moore, *Care of the Soul,* 183.
6. Ibid., 185.

Bryophytes

1. Nancy J. Turner, John Thomas, Barry F. Carlson, and Robert T. Ogilvie, *Ethnobotany of the Nitinaht Indians of Vancouver Island* (Victoria, Canada: British Columbia Provincial Museum, 1983), 58.
2. Erich Fromm, *The Anatomy of Human Destructiveness* (New York: Holt, Rinehart and Winston, 1973), 362–407.
3. Bruce H. Lipton, *The Honeymoon Effect: The Science of Creating Heaven on Earth* (Carlsbad, CA: Hay House, 2013), 77–78.
4. C. Louis Kervran and Michel Abehsera, *Biological Transmutations, and Their Applications in Chemistry, Physics, Biology, Ecology, Medicine, Nutrition, Agriculture, Geology* (Binghamton, NY: Swan House, 1972).

BIBLIOGRAPHY

Abenheimer, K. M. "The Ego as Subject." In *The Reality of the Psyche*. Edited by Joseph B. Wheelwright. New York: Putnam, 1968, 61–73.

American Psychiatric Association. *Diagnostic and Statistical Manual of Mental Disorders: DSM-5*. Washington, DC: American Psychiatric Association, 2013.

Bach, Edward. *Heal Thyself: An Explanation of the Real Cause and Cure of Disease*. London: C. W. Daniel, 1931.

Ball, Martin W. *Mushroom Wisdom: How Shamans Cultivate Spiritual Consciousness*. Oakland, CA: Ronin, 2006.

Bangen, Katherine J., Marianne Bergheim, Allison R. Kaup, Heline Mirzakhanian, Christina E. Wierenga, Dilip V. Jeste, and Lisa T. Eyler. "Brains of Optimistic Older Adults Respond Less to Fearful Faces." *Journal of Neuropsychiatry and Clinical Neurosciences* 26 (2: spring 2014), 155–63. doi:10.1176/appi.neuropsych.12090231.

Baring, Anne, and Jules Cashford. *The Myth of the Goddess: Evolution of an Image*. New York: Viking Arkana, 1991.

Barreto, Michael. "Astrology Affects the Yield of Shiitake Mushrooms." Aztro1.com. May 28, 2014. www.aztro1.com/research/biodynamic-mushroom-farming.htm.

Berendt, Joachim-Ernst. *The Third Ear: On Listening to the World*. Translated by Tim Nevill. Shaftesbury, UK: Element, 1988.

Blake, William. *The Marriage of Heaven and Hell*. 17932 object 14.

Bly, Robert. *A Little Book on the Human Shadow*. New York: HarperCollins, 1988.

Buhner, Stephen Harrod. *Plant Intelligence and the Imaginal Realm: Beyond the Doors of Perception into the Dreaming Earth*. Rochester, VT: Bear & Co., 2014.

Campbell, Joseph. *The Hero with a Thousand Faces*. New York: Pantheon, 1949.

Coan, James A., Hillary S. Schaefer, and Richard J. Davidson. "Lending a Hand: Social Regulation of the Neural Response to Threat," *Psychological Science* 17:12 (December 2006), 1032–39. doi:10.1111/j.1467-9280.2006.01832.x.

Decety, Jean, Jason M. Cowell, Kang Lee, Randa Mahasneh, Susan Malcolm-Smith, Bilge Selcuk, and Xinyue Zhou. "The Negative Association between

Religiousness and Children's Altruism across the World." *Current Biology* 25:22 (November 16, 2015), 2951–55. doi:10.1016/j.cub.2015.09.056.

Dessen, Sarah, and Nancy Brennan. *Lock and Key: A Novel*. New York: Viking, 2008.

Dias, Brian G., and Kerry J. Ressler. "Parental Olfactory Experience Influences Behavior and Neural Structure in Subsequent Generations." *Nature Neuroscience* 17 (2014), 89–96. doi:10.1038/nn.3594.

Didymus, Johnthomas. "Religious Fundamentalism Could Soon Be Treated as Mental Illness." Digital Journal, June 2, 2013, http://www.digitaljournal.com/article/351347.

Dodes, Lance M., and Zachary Dodes. *The Sober Truth: Debunking the Bad Science Behind 12-Step Programs and the Rehab Industry*. Boston: Beacon Press, 2014.

Einstein, Albert. *Cosmic Religion: With Other Opinions and Aphorisms*. New York: Covici-Friede, 1931.

Estés, Clarissa Pinkola. *Women Who Run with the Wolves: Myths and Stories of the Wild Woman Archetype*. New York: Ballantine, 1992.

Ferenczi, Sándor, Judith Dupont, Michael Balint, and Nicola Zarday Jackson. *The Clinical Diary of Sándor Ferenczi*. Cambridge, MA: Harvard University Press, 1995.

Filevich, Elisa, Martin Dresler, Timothy R. Brick, and Simone Kühn. "Metacognitive Mechanisms Underlying Lucid Dreaming." *The Journal of Neuroscience* 35 (3: January 21, 2015), 1082–88. doi:10.1523 /JNEUROSCI.3342-14.2015.

Fromm, Erich. *The Anatomy of Human Destructiveness*. New York: Holt, Rinehart and Winston, 1973.

Gershon, Michael D. *The Second Brain: The Scientific Basis of Gut Instinct and a Groundbreaking New Understanding of Nervous Disorders of the Stomach and Intestine*. New York: HarperCollins, 1998.

Graves, Julia. *The Language of Plants: A Guide to the Doctrine of Signatures*. Great Barrington, MA: Lindisfarne, 2012.

Gurdjieff, G. I. *Meetings with Remarkable Men*. Translated by A. R. Orage. New York: E. P. Dutton, 1963.

Hall, Nor. *The Moon and the Virgin: Reflections on the Archetypal Feminine*. New York: Harper & Row, 1980.

Harvey, Clare G., Andreas Korte, George Lewith, and Richard Gerber. *The Practitioner's Encyclopedia of Flower Remedies: The Definitive Guide to All Flower Essences, Their Making and Uses*. Philadelphia: Singing Dragon, 2015.

Heinrich, Clark. *Magic Mushrooms in Religion and Alchemy.* Rochester, VT: Park Street Press, 2002.

Hickey, Steve, and Hilary Roberts. *Tarnished Gold: The Sickness of Evidence-Based Medicine.* Lexington, KY: Newlyn Research Group, 2011.

Hillman, James. *Re-Visioning Psychology.* New York: Harper & Row, 1975.

Huxley, Thomas Henry. "On the Advisableness of Improving Natural Knowledge." 1866. In *Selected Essays and Addresses of Thomas Henry Huxley,* edited by Philo Melvyn Buck Jr. New York: Macmillan, 1910.

Irvin, J. R., and Jack Herer. *The Holy Mushroom: Evidence of Mushrooms in Judeo-Christianity.* Gnostic Media Research & Pub., 2008.

Jung, C. G. "The Aims of Psychotherapy." *The Collected Works of C. G. Jung, Vol. 16: The Practice of Psychotherapy.* New York: Panthcon, 1953.

———. *Archetypes and the Collective Unconscious.* Translated by R. F. C. Hull. Princeton, NJ: Princeton University Press, 1959.

———. *Dream Analysis: Notes of the Seminar Given in 1928–1930.* London: Routledge & Kegan Paul, 1984.

———. *Memories, Dreams, Reflections.* New York: Pantheon, 1963.

———. *The Undiscovered Self.* New York: Little, Brown, 1958.

Keen, Sam. *Fire in the Belly: On Being a Man.* New York: Bantam, 1991.

Kervran, C. Louis, and Michel Abehsera. *Biological Transmutations, and Their Applications in Chemistry, Physics, Biology, Ecology, Medicine, Nutrition, Agriculture, Geology.* Binghamton, NY: Swan House, 1972.

Kolbert, Elizabeth. "Thomas Friedman: Hope for a Hot, Flat and Crowded World." *Yale Environment 360.* October 9, 2008.

Lazaris. "Working with Your Shadow I: An Imperative on the Spiritual Path." *New Moon Rising* 42 (March–April 1996), http://www.nmrjournal.com/zine/archive/issues/42/444.htm.

Lipton, Bruce H. *The Honeymoon Effect: The Science of Creating Heaven on Earth.* Carlsbad, CA: Hay House, 2013.

Louv, Richard. "Children and Nature Movement: How a Movement Is Forming and How You Can Get Involved." March 2008. http://richardlouv.com/books/last-child/children-nature-movement/.

———. *Last Child in the Woods: Saving Our Children from Nature-Deficit Disorder.* Chapel Hill, NC: Algonquin Books, 2006.

Master, Sarah L., Naomi I. Eisenberger, Shelley E. Taylor, Bruce D. Naliboff, David Shirinyan, and Matthew D. Lieberman. "A Picture's Worth: Partner Photographs Reduce Experimentally Induced Pain." *Psychological Science* 20:11 (2009), 1316–18. doi:10.1111/j.1467-9280.2009.02444.x.

Moore, Thomas. *Care of the Soul: A Guide for Cultivating Depth and Sacredness in Everyday Life.* New York: Harper Collins, 1992.

O'Mara, Erin M., James K. McNulty, and B. R. Karney. "Positively Biased Appraisals in Everyday Life: When Do They Benefit Mental Health and When Do They Harm It?" *Journal of Personality and Social Psychology* 101 (3: September 2011), 415–32. doi:10.1037/a0023332.

Orwell, George, Sonia Orwell, and Ian Angus. *The Collected Essays, Journalism, and Letters of George Orwell.* New York: Harcourt, Brace, 1968.

Peck, R. C. "Psychological Developments in the Second Half of Life." In *Middle Age and Aging: A Reader in Social Psychology,* edited by Bernice L. Neugarten. Chicago: University of Chicago Press, 1968.

Pedersen, Susanne S., Pedro A. Lemos, Priya R. van Vooren, Tommy K. K. Liu, Joost Daemen, Ruud A. M. Erdman, Pieter C. Smits, et al. "Type D Personality Predicts Death or Myocardial Infarction after Bare Metal Stent or Sirolimus-Eluting Stent Implantation." *Journal of the American College of Cardiology* 44 (5:2004), 997–1001. doi:10.1016/j.jacc.2004.05.064.

Plotkin, Bill. *Soulcraft: Crossing into the Mysteries of Nature and Psyche.* Novato, CA: New World Library, 2003.

Reddy, Sumathi. "A Perfect Dose of Pessimism." *Wall Street Journal.* August 5, 2014.

Richo, David. *How to Be an Adult: A Handbook on Psychological and Spiritual Integration,* New York: Paulist Press, 2002.

Rohr, Richard. *Falling Upward: A Spirituality for the Two Halves of Life.* San Francisco: Jossey-Bass, 2011.

Rush, John A. *The Mushroom in Christian Art: The Identity of Jesus in the Development of Christianity.* Berkeley, CA: North Atlantic Books, 2011.

Sardello, Robert J. *Facing the World with Soul: The Reimagination of Modern Life.* New York: HarperPerennial, 1994.

Schrödinger, Erwin. *Science and Humanism; Physics in Our Time.* Cambridge, UK: Cambridge University Press, 1951.

Schwarz, Jack. *It's Not What You Eat but What Eats You.* Berkeley, CA: Celestial Arts, 1988.

Segerstrom, Suzanne C. *Breaking Murphy's Law: How Optimists Get What They Want from Life—and Pessimists Can Too.* New York: Guilford Press, 2006.

Stevens, José. *Transforming Your Dragons: Turning Personality Fear Patterns into Personal Power.* Santa Fe, NM: Bear and Co., 1994.

Susanne S. Pedersen, Pedro A. Lemos, Priya R. van Vooren, Tommy K. K. Liu, Joost Daemen, Ruud A. M. Erdman, Pieter C. Smits, Patrick W. J. C.

Serruys, and Ron T. van Domburg. "Type D Personality Predicts Death or Myocardial Infarction after Bare Metal Stent or Sirolimus-Eluting Stent Implantation." *Journal of the American College of Cardiology* 44 (5:2004), 997–1001. doi:10.1016/j.jacc.2004.05.064.

Turner, Nancy J., John Thomas, Barry F. Carlson, and Robert T. Ogilvie. *Ethnobotany of the Nitinaht Indians of Vancouver Island.* Victoria, Canada: British Columbia Provincial Museum, 1983.

Twentyman, Ralph. *The Science and Art of Healing.* Edinburgh: Floris Books, 1989.

Vermeulen, Frans. *Fungi: Kingdom Fungi.* Haarlem, Netherlands: Emryss, 2007.

Whitmont, Edward C. *Psyche and Substance: Essays on Homeopathy in the Light of Jungian Psychology.* Berkeley, CA: North Atlantic Books, 1980.

———. *The Symbolic Quest: Basic Concepts of Analytical Psychology.* Princeton, NJ: Princeton University Press, 1969.

Wood, Matthew. *The Book of Herbal Wisdom: Using Plants as Medicines.* Berkeley, CA: North Atlantic Books, 1997.

———. *Vitalism: The History of Herbalism, Homeopathy, and Flower Essences.* Berkeley, CA: North Atlantic, 2000.

Zilvar, Tomas, and Radeq Brousil. "The Mushroom Whisperer." *Vice,* October 27, 2011. www.vice.com/read/Vaclav-Halek-makes-mushroom-music.

Zimecki, M. "The Lunar Cycle: Effects on Human and Animal Behavior and Physiology." *Postępy higieny i medycyny doświadczalnej* (Warsaw) 60 (2006): 1–7.

RESOURCES

Carlson, Richard, and Benjamin Shield. *Handbook for the Soul.* Boston: Little, Brown, 1995.

Graves, Julia. *The Language of Plants: A Guide to the Doctrine of Signatures.* Great Barrington, MA: Lindisfarne, 2012.

Gurdjieff, G. I. *Meetings with Remarkable Men.* Translated by A. R. Orage. New York: E. P. Dutton, 1963.

Heinrich, Clark. *Magic Mushrooms in Religion and Alchemy.* Rochester, VT: Park Street Press, 2002.

Irvin, J. R., and Jack Herer. *The Holy Mushroom: Evidence of Mushrooms in Judeo-Christianity.* Gnostic Media Research & Pub., 2008.

Jesso, James W. *Decomposing the Shadow: Lessons from the Psilocybin Mushroom.* Calgary: SoulsLantern, 2014.

Kervran, C. Louis, and Michel Abehsera. *Biological Transmutations, and Their Applications in Chemistry, Physics, Biology, Ecology, Medicine, Nutrition, Agriculture, Geology.* Binghamton, NY: Swan House, 1972.

Leader, Darian, and David Corfield. *Why People Get Sick: Exploring the Mind-Body Connection.* New York: Pegasus, 2008.

Moore, Thomas. *Care of the Soul: A Guide for Cultivating Depth and Sacredness in Everyday Life.* New York: Harper Collins, 1992.

Peck, R. C. "Psychological Developments in the Second Half of Life." In *Middle Age and Aging: A Reader in Social Psychology,* edited by Bernice L. Neugarten. Chicago: University of Chicago Press, 1968.

Plotkin, Bill. *Soulcraft: Crossing into the Mysteries of Nature and Psyche.* Novato, CA: New World Library, 2003.

———. *Wild Mind: A Field Guide to the Human Psyche.* Novato, CA: New World Library, 2013.

Rush, John A. *The Mushroom in Christian Art: The Identity of Jesus in the Development of Christianity.* Berkeley, CA: North Atlantic Books, 2011.

Sardello, Robert J. *Facing the World with Soul: The Reimagination of Modern Life.* New York: HarperPerennial, 1994.

Schwarz, Jack. *It's Not What You Eat but What Eats You.* Berkeley, CA: Celestial Arts, 1988.

Smith, Daniel B. *Muses, Madmen, and Prophets: Rethinking the History, Science, and Meaning of Auditory Hallucination*. New York: Penguin Press, 2007.

Stevens, José. *Transforming Your Dragons: Turning Personality Fear Patterns into Personal Power*. Santa Fe, NM: Bear and Co., 1994.

Zweig, Connie, and Steve Wolf. *Romancing the Shadow: A Guide to Soul Work for a Vital, Authentic Life*. New York: Ballantine, 1999.

Recommended Fungi Poetry and Short Stories

Chadwick, Kelly, and Renée Roehl. *Decomposition: An Anthology of Fungi-Inspired Poems*. Sandpoint, ID: Lost Horse Press, 2010.

Grey, Orrin, and Silvia Moreno-Garcia. *Fungi*. Vancouver, Canada: Innsmouth Free Press, 2012.

Prairie Deva Mushroom Essences

All mushroom essences are available in stock bottles. The retail price is US$12.95; minimum order is US$100.

Kits containing all 48 essences retail for US$495, with shipping available throughout Canada and the United States. Flower essence practitioners may request a 20 percent discount. Visa and MasterCard are accepted.

The email address for orders is scents@telusplanet.net. You may also order by mail: Self Heal Distributing, Box 95008, Whyte PO, Edmonton, AB, Canada, T6E 0E5.

Visit www.selfhealdistributing.com for a full list of essences and books.

INDEX

Dissolution, 4
Distinction, 44, 45, 233
Divinity, 89, 233
Divorce, 125, 127, 233
DMT, 40, 233
DNA, 200, 201, 233
Dodes, Lance, 163
Dogs, 115, 117, 119, 233
Dog stinkhorn (*Mutinus elegans*),
    166–70, 230, 231, 232, 234, 235,
    236, 237, 242
Dolichousnea longissima. See Usnea
Doors of perception, 186, 187, 233
Dopamine, 25, 214, 233
Dreams, 48, 49, 77, 78, 79, 115, 117,
    125, 127, 233. *See also* Lucid
    dreaming
Drew, Nancy, 185
Drowning, 128, 129, 233
Dubay, Eric, 131
Dupuytren's contracture, 135, 137, 233

E

Earthquakes, 115, 117–18, 233
Earth star (*Geastrum triplex*), 162–65,
    230, 232, 234, 235, 236, 237, 241
Eczema, 150, 152, 233
Edison, Thomas A., 150
Egotism, 44, 233
Einstein, Albert, 197
Elder wisdom, 104, 106–7, 233
Elf cup. *See* Green elf cup
Emotional flexibility, 73–75, 233
Empathy, 19, 21, 166, 169, 234
Empedocles, 192
Empty nest syndrome, 73, 75, 234
Enlightenment, 65, 66, 234
Enoki (*Flammulina velutipes*), 151, 244
Entitlement, 50, 234
Envy, 53, 55, 60, 61, 181–84, 234
Epimendes, 186–87
Equality, 205, 206, 234

Erhard, Werner, 196
Erotic parts, 176, 234
Escapism, 162, 163, 234
Estés, Clarissa Pinkola, 216
Euthanasia, 209, 210, 234
Evidence-based medicine, 92, 93, 234
Exhaustion, 158, 159, 234
Expansion and contraction, 135, 136–
    38, 232, 234
Exposure, 151, 234
Extroversion, 162, 163, 234
Exuberance, 81

F

Fairy ring (*Marasmius oreades*), 140–43,
    231, 232, 234, 235, 236, 237, 238
Faith, 77, 234
Family, 117, 234
Fast, Alexia, 53
Fasting, 88, 90, 234
Fear, 33, 34, 109, 111, 130, 132, 200,
    201, 234
    of success, 69, 70, 234
    of water, 79, 234
Feelings, 115, 116, 234
Femininity, 81, 82, 185, 234
Ferenczi, Sándor, 93
Fermentation, 5–6
Fertility, 140, 141, 234
Ficino, Marsilio, 92
Fitzgerald, F. Scott, 73
Flammulina populicola. See Velvet foot
Flammulina velutipes. See Enoki
Flexibility, 29, 31, 104, 181, 184, 234
Floods, 77, 78, 234
Flower essences, xix
Fly agaric (*Amanita muscaria*), 135–39,
    230, 231, 232, 233, 235, 236, 237,
    238, 239, 240, 244
Flying, 171, 172
Fomes fomentarius. See Tinder conk
Fomitopsis cajanderi. See Rosy conk

ABOUT THE AUTHOR

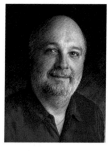 Robert Dale Rogers has been an herbalist for over forty years. He has a Bachelor of Science from the University of Alberta, where he is an assistant clinical professor in family medicine. He taught plant medicine, including herbology and flower essences, at MacEwan University for ten years, and presently, in the Earth Spirit Medicine Program at the Northern Star College in Edmonton.

Robert is past chair of the Alberta Natural Health Agricultural Network and Community Health Council of Capital Health. He is a Fellow of the International College of Nutrition, past chair of the medicinal mushroom committee of the North American Mycological Association, and on the editorial boards of the *International Journal of Medicinal Mushrooms* and *Discovery Phytomedicine*. Robert cohosts The Alberta Herb Gathering (www.herbgatheringalberta.com), held every other year.

He lives on Millcreek Ravine in Edmonton with his beautiful and talented wife, Laurie Szott-Rogers, and an out-of-control cat, Ceres. You can email him at scents@telusplanet.net or visit www.selfhealdistributing.com.

ABOUT
NORTH ATLANTIC BOOKS

North Atlantic Books (NAB) is an independent, nonprofit publisher committed to a bold exploration of the relationships between mind, body, spirit, and nature. Founded in 1974, NAB aims to nurture a holistic view of the arts, sciences, humanities, and healing. To make a donation or to learn more about our books, authors, events, and newsletter, please visit www.northatlanticbooks.com.